The New Fertility

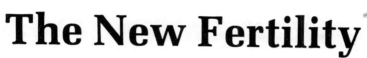

The New Fertility

**A guide to modern medical treatment
for childless couples**

GRAHAM H. BARKER, FRCS, MRCOG

Foreword by Patrick Steptoe, FRCS, FRCOG

Illustrations by Jennie Smith

Adamson Books
London

Text copyright © 1986 Graham H. Barker
Illustrations copyright © 1986 Adamson Books

Published by Adamson Books
6 Foxbourne Road
London SW17 8EW

Cover design by Jonathan Raimes and Dave Allen
Book design by Nicky Adamson

British Library Cataloguing in Publication Data
Barker, Graham H.
    The new fertility: a guide to modern
    medical treatment for childless couples.
    1. Infertility—Treatment
    I. Title.
    616.6'9206   RC889

    ISBN 0-948543-15-9
    ISBN 0-948543-10-8 Pbk

Typeset by Vantage Photosetting Co Ltd,
Eastleigh and London
Printed in Great Britain by the Hollen Street Press

Contents

Foreword

The investigations and treatments now available to a couple who have difficulty in having a child have been greatly advanced and improved over the past decade. It is not easy for every couple to understand the normal processes involved in conception and the many ways in which problems occur, and their necessary remedies. Doctors and other workers involved with fertility treatments are unable to give each couple a complete and thorough explanation of the complex processes and treatments at each consultation. Yet a couple's understanding of these processes and treatments will greatly help both themselves and their doctors and, of course, reduce stress and anxiety on all sides. This book aims to explain fertility problems and their treatment in a helpful, sympathetic and detailed way, and I hope its readers will greatly benefit from the understanding they derive from it.

PATRICK STEPTOE FRCS, FRCOG
Director, Bourn Hall Clinic,
Bourn, Cambridge

Preface

Any couple who, either temporarily or permanently, are unable to have children when they wish to face many problems—emotional, psychological, and possibly medical. They frequently experience frustration, anger, and bewilderment at the relative complexity of infertility, its investigation and possible treatment. Apart from having to come to terms with their problem—the usual reaction of any couple to the possibility that they are unable to have children is 'Why me? Why us?'—the couple will also meet with the sometimes formidable problem of understanding what the doctor is doing to find out what, if anything, is wrong, and to help them conceive.

The aim of this book is to answer as many questions about infertility as possible, and also to dispel apprehension and encourage a more enlightened approach to the problems of investigating and treating infertility. This is a subject both fascinating and frustrating, and it may well intrigue those who are not infertile themselves but wish to know more about it.

However, this book is primarily designed for couples who are just starting their 'infertility investigations' or those who are perhaps thinking that they might need medical help. Therefore, instead of starting the book with a massive lecture on normal anatomy and the physiology of conception (which would possibly confuse and probably bore you), I am going to plunge straight into the subject, just as you would with your doctor, and try to explain the basics as we go through the book. I hope to guide you along the path that the 'average' series of infertility investigations and treatments takes—so that with each chapter your knowledge increases gradually. We will explore some rare sidetracks along our path, and certain areas, where there are important points to explain and emphasize, will be covered more than once.

Your doctor will endeavour to carry out your investigations with thoroughness, skill and tact, and with economy of time and effort all round. Likewise, he or she will rely to some extent on your understanding and cooperation: indeed, the chances of a successful outcome are increased if a couple understand thoroughly what information is required and why.

In infertility, unlike illness, people consult a doctor for assistance when they are essentially healthy, and frequently they take great interest in the tests and procedures which they hope will eventually give the clue to solving their problem; they also develop a different relationship with the doctor from that which arises in treating illness.

The doctor who tries to explain to couples both the basis of fertility and the means of testing it during a few precious minutes in the clinic faces an uphill task. At the end of the day his or her pad will be covered with little diagrams of Fallopian tubes and menstrual cycles, and however hard he or she has tried to be clear, much confusion will remain. Similarly, every doctor finds that problems can be discussed in much greater and more satisfying depth if couples have even a minor degree of subject knowledge; each consultation then becomes more fruitful and stimulating for all concerned.

I wanted to write this book right from my early training in gynaecology—ever since, in fact, I first tried to explain to infertile patients what our complex tests and treatments involved and meant. It was originally published in the United States of America, and has now been fully revised and updated, with new illustrations, for publication in the United Kingdom and the rest of the English-speaking world; it is to the directors of Adamson Books, Nicky and Stephen Adamson, that I record my sincere gratitude as well as the thanks of many readers now and in the future.

GRAHAM BARKER
London, 1986

Introduction

It is estimated that some 10 per cent of all couples in Europe experience a period of infertility. As many as 8 per cent of marriages remain childless after ten years. It may be true that we live in an age where the overproduction of children is not encouraged, that there is a growing acceptance that the careers of certain couples might preclude children, and that consequently the emphasis on parenthood as the natural product of pair bonding has declined. Nevertheless, the desire to produce children is deeply rooted in biological instinct and represents for most people a means of emotional fulfilment and a natural expression of love. The couple who cannot have children when they want to often feel enormous sadness and frustration. Added to this, social and family pressures are often still very strong; the newly-weds of many societies (even grossly overpopulated ones) still commence their married life among ancient fertility rites (e.g., rose-petal and rice throwing) and prayers for fecundity. History is littered with stories and events which revolve around childbirth and inheritance, and the fortunes of all monarchies, however powerful, have rested upon the production of suitable heirs. The wives of Henry VIII had strong views on this subject, and like it or not, the average young couple today will need a thick skin before announcing to the potential grandparents that they have decided not to embark upon a family.

Overcoming stress

The couple, therefore, who find themselves unable to conceive will frequently be under stress and a mixed feeling of guilt and mistrust may pervade. To minimize the build-up of stress—which can only aggravate the problem—it is essential that they should, as early as possible, seek and obtain expert advice in order to investigate the cause of their difficulty and, if necessary, to receive appropriate treatment.

No discussion of fertility can leave aside the connections between marital stability and parenthood. On the one hand, many marriages have been stabilized by the addition of a child (though parenthood is by no means a panacea for all marital ills). On the other hand, psychological stresses produced by discord between the partners can delay conception—in obvious ways such as by interrupting the pattern and frequency of intercourse, and more subtle ways, such as an unconscious, anxiety-induced inhibition of conception. It is difficult to find an explanation for the psychological causes of infertility, but they do seem to exist: many couples who have experienced serious marital discord accompanied by infertility have found no problem in conceiving during subsequent periods of relative calm and relaxation.

Please do not think that I am trying to suggest that all problems of infertility are 'in the mind'. They are not, and all infertile couples should be properly and scientifically investigated if they so desire. Nevertheless the psychological aspect is extremely important in some cases—as most people working in this field will testify. Many couples conceive soon after infertility investigations have begun, perhaps because they can relax in the reassuring knowledge that their problem is being addressed. All practitioners have stories to tell of couples 'barren' for many years and who suddenly find themselves proud parents. It is also common to find normal couples who have not used contraception and whose children are well spaced out, with several years between each.

Time factors

There is much variety in the speed with which couples are able to produce children, and this is not surprising when we consider the many complex factors and interactions required to initiate and sustain a pregnancy. Some women become pregnant almost as soon as contraceptive precautions are abandoned, while some couples wait several years before the first child is born. Mutual and individual fertility varies throughout life but, in general, a woman's fertility tends to decline towards the end of her reproductive years, particularly after the age of 40, although pregnancies in women approaching 50 and even beyond are occasionally reported. The pattern in men is not so well defined and a man's reproductive life may well extend into very old age indeed.

Potency and fertility

There is an important distinction to be drawn here between infertility, the inability of a woman to conceive or of a man to father a child, and impotence, which is a man's inability to perform the sexual act. Although impotence may well be associated with infertility it must be emphasized that a man might easily be infertile and never have any problems of impotence. Infertile men and women may well enjoy a satisfactory and normal sex life but without, of course, conception taking place. Sadly there are many who mistakenly think that if a man cannot father a child he is probably impotent, and in some way 'less than a man'. This is usually completely wrong: many potent men with highly active sex lives are completely surprised to discover that they may well have been infertile for many years.

Unfortunately, such misguided associations between impotence and infertility may well give the couple who have difficulty conceiving immediate feelings of inferiority and guilt, which frequently discourage the man, at least, from seeking advice and assistance. It cannot be emphasized too strongly that, whereas impotence may be a problem for some infertile couples, the vast majority of those seeking advice from doctors have perfectly normal and satisfying sexual relationships.

What is normal?

So what do we mean by fertility, subfertility and infertility? These are rather imprecise terms to describe the variation from couples who conceive quickly and easily, through those who experience difficulties requiring medical assistance, to those who after extensive investigation and treatment remain childless.

Fertility, of course, can be temporarily interrupted— e.g., by the use of contraceptives, in which case it usually returns after their use is stopped—and so these terms are only applicable at particular times. Hospital departments dealing with this subject may well be called 'fertility centres' or 'fertility clinics', 'infertility clinics', or even 'subfertility clinics'. All these terms are relative and without qualification do not mean a great deal.

When should a couple seek advice? It is difficult to say precisely. There are no strict rules, but most doctors advise that a couple should have intercourse without the use of contraceptives for 12 to 18 months at least before being concerned that the woman has not become pregnant. However, one can see immediately that if for instance, a woman aged around 35 or more wishes to conceive, then she and her partner should perhaps try for only a year before seeking advice. On the whole it is better to seek medical opinion earlier rather than later, and if a couple come forward too early the doctor can always advise a further spell of trying before commencing investigations.

Health and fertility

Couples who wish to start a family should try to be as healthy as possible at the time of conception. Both partners should eat a healthy, balanced diet and before pregnancy a woman should avoid being overweight. Obesity in pregnancy can cause a variety of problems and many women find the extra weight is difficult to lose after their babies are born. However, avoid becoming too thin as well—this can affect fertility if taken to extremes (see p. 30).

A woman should also ensure that she is immune from rubella (German measles) so that when she becomes pregnant the longed-for baby is not put at risk from a rubella infection—which can cause blindness, deafness, mental retardation and cleft palate. The family doctor can check with a blood test to see if a woman is already immune (many will have been immunized at school or will have contracted the disease in childhood), and if she is not immune the doctor can immunize her with a simple injection.

Both partners should avoid excessive intakes of alcohol. Excess alcohol taken during the pregnancy may damage the developing baby. Both partners should also stop smoking. Smoking in pregnancy can cause growth problems in the baby, and men especially may find their fertility suppressed by excessive smoking and drinking. Both partners, especially the woman, should avoid taking drugs of any kind at conception and in early pregnancy unless advised to do so by a doctor.

Exercise on a regular basis is a helpful component of healthy living, but excessively hard exercise may affect fertility—in particular ovulation may be suppressed in women who work exceptionally hard at athletic pursuits. Again if in any doubt, consult a doctor.

1

Sex and subfertility

Technical problems with sex

In this chapter we shall look at some of the reasons why perfectly fertile couples may experience difficulty in having a baby. Most of these are to do with sex in one way or another, and for the purposes of this book we can think of them as 'technical problems' with sex. Some consist of difficulties with the sexual act itself, and may be caused, for example, by premature ejaculation or impotence in the man, or by pain experienced by the woman during intercourse; but others are concerned with the frequency and timing of intercourse and are not restricted to couples with unhappy sex lives, as we shall see. Couples may enjoy fulfilling sex and yet fail to conceive because they are making love too infrequently or at the wrong time. On the other hand, it is certainly true to say that couples do not need to have an exciting sex life in order to achieve a pregnancy. Technical problems, whether they relate to specific sexual difficulties or to the timing of intercourse, are very often easily rectified, and for obvious reasons the investigating doctor must eliminate any problems relating to sex before proceeding on to more complicated tests.

At this stage the doctor will already have established that the couple have spent a reasonable time trying to produce a child before coming foward for help. The next thing he or she will want to do is to make sure that both partners appreciate the normal requirements for fertilization and conception. (I shall be covering these requirements during the course of this chapter to illustrate how some technical problems arise; meanwhile the physiological elements of reproduction are given in diagrammatic form in the illustrations opposite.) A very

The reproductive organs

Male anatomy

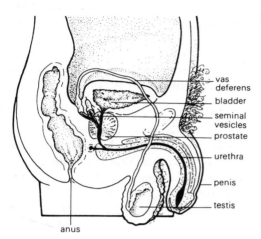

vas deferens
bladder
seminal vesicles
prostate
urethra
penis
testis
anus

Spermatazoon

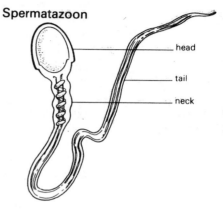

head
tail
neck

Female anatomy

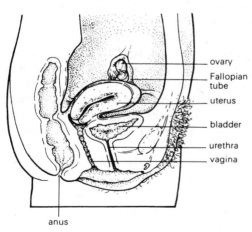

ovary
Fallopian tube
uterus
bladder
urethra
vagina
anus

Ovum

nucleus
corona radiata
zona pellucida

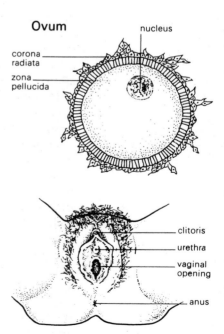

clitoris
urethra
vaginal opening
anus

External genitalia

small but ever-present proportion of infertile couples can have their problem solved by a simple explanation of the normal requirements. At the very extreme end of this group are couples who are not having normal sexual intercourse—with true failure of technique. It is not unknown for a doctor to discover that a couple have been practising rectal intercourse, for example. Such cases are relatively rare; it is much more common, however, that couples have not appreciated the importance of having intercourse reasonably frequently and, more importantly, at the right time of the woman's menstrual cycle.

Frequency of intercourse

Quite obviously, if a couple is having very infrequent sexual intercourse then the chances of conception remain low. Very occasionally couples will seek help from their doctor, and when asked will reveal that intercourse may take place perhaps only once a month or even once every two months. Work schedules in particular can often interfere with the frequency of intercourse, with one or other partner being out of town or abroad for long periods, or perhaps away with the armed forces. No one can lay down rules for the frequency of intercourse beyond certain loose guidelines, but many couples can achieve conception simply by changing their schedule to allow for more sex at the most advantageous time.

Incidentally, in the course of asking the couple about frequency of intercourse, the doctor may discover that immediately after sex the woman performs vigorous vaginal douching. This practice (which is fairly rare, especially nowadays) may well reduce the chances of conception; indeed, in some primitive societies a combination of vaginal douching and strenuous physical activity, such as running, is used immediately after intercourse as a feeble form of contraception. Let me say immediately, however, that this technique is by no means reliable, and should not be contemplated by anyone as a serious method of contraception! The reasons for the immediate postcoital washing, bathing or douching may go beyond simple vaginal hygiene; tactful questioning by the doctor may shed light on the woman's attitude towards sex in general, and in some cases may reveal that she equates the sex act with something that is generally unclean and dirty.

Further questioning may disclose some strain in the sexual relationship of the couple, producing the tension referred to on p. 10.

It may appear from what I have just said that something of a cross-examination is going on, but this should not be the case at all. A good doctor is sensitive to the fact that answering intimate questions about one's sex life does not come easily to many people, and will not conduct the investigations in the manner of an interrogation. Couples who may feel uncomfortable at the thought of talking about their sex life should remember that the doctor asks such questions as a routine, and is interested in the couple's replies only insofar as they are relevant to the job of solving their problems.

Timing of intercourse

We have already seen that the childless couple should have sex with a certain minimum frequency; however, it is extremely important that they also have it at the time of the month when the woman is most likely to be fertile. This is a matter of only a day or two. We do not know for sure how long the spermatozoa in the male ejaculate remain viable (able to fertilize the female egg), but a round figure of between 24 and 48 hours seems reasonable. The life of the egg cell (ovum) is also relatively short—perhaps only 10–12 hours, or sometimes up to 24 hours. It therefore follows that for conception to occur, intercourse must take place within a day or so of ovulation—the release of the ovum from the ovary. However, before going into more detail, I will give a summary of the events leading up to conception.

How conception is achieved

After a woman has had her menstrual period, the pituitary gland in the brain secretes hormones which stimulate the ripening of an ovum in one of her ovaries (they usually alternate each month), and under the influence of these hormones, the ripe ovum will be released by the ovary. This occurs at approximately the midpoint of the menstrual cycle, although the timing varies, depending on the length of each woman's period (see p. 46). At the end of the Fallopian tubes are finger-like projections (fimbriae) which play over the surface of the ovary.

After its release the ovum is grasped by the fimbriae and

Menstrual cycle

1 Pituitary gland hormones (LH and FSH) stimulate the growth of an egg follicle in the ovary.

2 As the follicle ripens (A), the ovaries produce the hormones progesterone and oestrogen, which stimulate the growth of the lining of the uterus (endometrium). At ovulation (B), the egg (ovum) bursts out of the follicle, is collected by the fimbriae and passes into the fallopian tube.
The empty follicle closes and becomes a corpus luteum (C), producing oestrogen and rising amounts of progesterone. Unless pregnancy occurs, it gradually degenerates.

3 In preparation for receiving an ovum, the endometrium thickens in the first half of the cycle (a). In the second half, (b) glands secrete a rich nutritive substance.

4 Under the influence of ovarian and pituitary hormones, changes also occur in the cervix, vagina

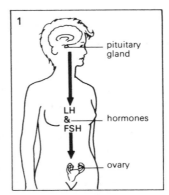

pituitary gland

LH & FSH — hormones

ovary

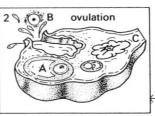

2   B   **ovulation**

A   C

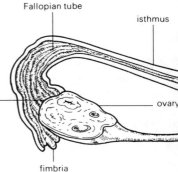

Fallopian tube

isthmus

ovary

fimbria

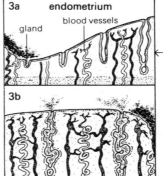

3a   **endometrium**
gland   blood vessels

3b

The reproductive cycle

The process by which a woman's body prepares itself for fertilization and pregnancy is complex. However a clear understanding of the mechanisms involved is vital for those seeking treatment for infertility.

and fallopian tubes. The actual release of the ovum is stimulated by a surge of LH (luteinizing hormone) from the pituitary gland. NB The illustration (right) is approximately life size.

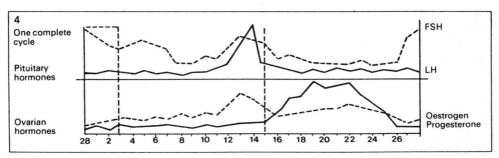

4
One complete cycle

Pituitary hormones

Ovarian hormones

FSH

LH

Oestrogen
Progesterone

28   2   4   6   8   10   12   14   16   18   20   22   24   26

Fertilization and implantation

5 During normal sexual intercourse, several million sperm are deposited high inside the vagina, leaving a pool of semen near the cervix.

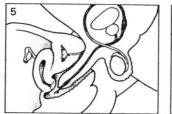

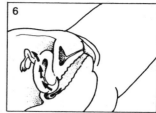

6 The sperm travel up into the uterus and then to the fallopian tubes. An ovum will be waiting there if ovulation has occurred.

7 For fertilization to occur, one spermatozoon must enter the ovum (a). Afterwards, the ovum begins to divide into a 2-cell stage (b), then 4, 8, 16 and so on. After about 3 days the ovum, now called a blastocyst (c), reaches the uterus, where it remains free for several days (d).

About 7 days after fertilization, the blastocyst implants into the thickened, glandular endometrium (e), obtaining nutrients from it until the placenta takes over.

8 In the ovary, the corpus luteum enlarges to maintain the pregnancy by producing oestrogen and progesterone. After about 8 weeks the placenta manufactures these hormones.

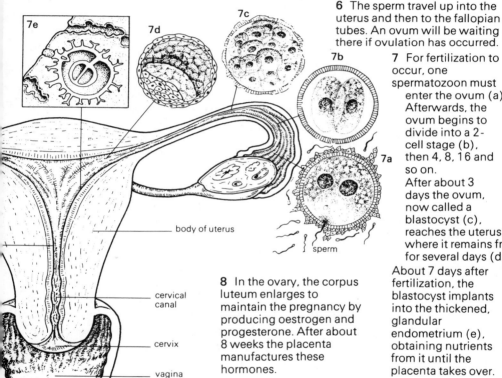

body of uterus

cervical canal

cervix

vagina

sperm

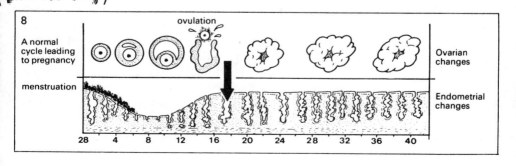

8

A normal cycle leading to pregnancy

ovulation

menstruation

Ovarian changes

Endometrial changes

28 4 8 12 16 20 24 28 32 36 40

conducted into the Fallopian tube; it passes down the narrow bore of the tube towards the uterus. During normal sexual intercourse a large number of spermatozoa in the male ejaculate (up to 500 million or more) are deposited high inside the vagina, adjacent to the neck of the womb (cervix). The spermatozoa then pass through a plug of mucus situated at the entrance to the womb, in the cervix. During this passage the spermatozoa are cleansed of certain proteins and the fluid in which they have travelled. This change is part of an essential process known as 'capacitation', which helps the spermatozoa to penetrate the ovum when they meet it in the Fallopian tube. Through uterine contractions the spermatozoa are conducted to the top of the uterus and make their way along the Fallopian tube towards the ovum. When viable spermatozoa meet a viable ovum, fertilization may occur, which is the penetration of the ovum by one spermatozoon. After fertilization, no further spermatozoon is able to enter.

The fertilized ovum remains in the tube and begins to divide, first into two cells, then four, then eight, then sixteen, and so on. This process takes about three days, after which the little bundle of cells, looking rather like a mulberry, migrates down the tube into the uterus. This mass of cells, called a morula, becomes pressed against its outer membrane, leaving a fluid–filled space. At this stage of development it is called a blastocyst. The blastocyst begins to implant itself into the glandular lining of the uterus on the sixth or seventh day after ovulation. The most usual position is at the top and back of the uterus, although it may implant in other parts.

After the release of the ovum from the ovary at the midpoint of the menstrual cycle, the lining of the uterus becomes ready for the arrival of a fertilized ovum. Stimulated by hormones from the ovary, it becomes thickened and more glandular. It also produces nourishing secretions without which the little embryo cannot survive. (This second half of the menstrual cycle is frequently referred to as the secretory phase.) As the pregnancy progresses and the embryo and its membranes enlarge, further hormones to sustain these processes are produced by the follicle within the ovary from which the ovum was released; the follicle has expanded and while it secretes these hormones it is known as the corpus luteum.

As mentioned earlier, the whole process leading to conception depends above all on one fundamental, and that is the timing of intercourse. Obviously, there are numerous other factors which must be fulfilled, but intercourse must take place on or around the time that the ovum is released, otherwise viable spermatozoa will not meet a viable ovum in the Fallopian tube. It is generally recommended that the man should abstain from intercourse and masturbation for two or three days in order to maximize the number of sperm in his ejaculate before the couple have intercourse around the midcycle time. Most women ovulate at about the 12th to 14th day of the cycle. This means that, counting the first day of proper bleeding in the woman's menstruation as day 1 of the cycle, a period of abstinence should be exercised from, say, day 6 or 7, with intercourse taking place on day 10 and after a gap of, say, 48 hours, again on day 12, and maybe on day 14 or 15.

When should you have sex?

This is only very general advice, based on a regular menstrual cycle of 28 days. The first thing to remember is that the length of the menstrual cycle (and thus the time of ovulation) varies from one woman to another and may also vary in the same woman from month to month— maybe only a few days' difference, but in some cases up to a week or more. Besides, many couples would find it awkward and possibly unnatural to have intercourse on a timetable as rigid as a British Airways flight schedule! However, while the foregoing is only a very rough guide, it is obvious that couples having intercourse only at the beginning or end of the menstrual cycle are unlikely to conceive. The timing of intercourse and the use of temperature charts is discussed further on pp. 45–47.

Most other mammals do not have this timing problem, in that they mate only at the time the female is likely to conceive (e.g., dogs, horses); moreover, in some species (cats, rabbits, ferrets) the female does not produce an ovum until the spermatozoa have arrived safely in the uterus, while in others she stores the spermatozoa successfully until the ovum has been released. Interestingly, however, there is some evidence that human females, following emotional and other stimuli, can produce ova at times other than midcycle. It is not uncommon for couples who practice the 'safe period' as a means of contraception (avoiding intercourse during mid-cycle when the ovum is likely to be viable and in the Fallopian tube) to be surprised by a pregnancy ensuing, and this can only be explained by ovulation occurring much earlier or later than expected.

Positions for intercourse

Couples sometimes ask whether any particular position during intercourse is more likely to result in pregnancy. While the general answer is no, it is important for the seminal fluid to be deposited near the cervix, and a position which allows a reasonable degree of penetration of the penis into the vagina is therefore desirable. The size of the man's penis is generally unimportant, again so long as penetration is achieved. The vagina is an elastic muscular sheath which can expand to accommodate different-sized male organs.

It is sometimes recommended that the woman should lie on her back for some minutes after sex, perhaps with a cushion underneath her buttocks to allow the sperm to collect near the cervix. On the other hand, some women whose uteruses are angled backwards rather than forwards (known as retroversion, and found in about one in every four or five women) experience discomfort when lying on their backs during intercourse. This may be relieved if the man lies on his back with the woman on top, allowing the uterus to flop forwards out of the way of the penis.

Perhaps the most important aspect of different positions is that by creating variety they enhance enjoyment of sex; in this way they can contribute to a happy sexual relationship, which is beneficial to men and women trying to create an environment suitable for conception.

Contrary to some people's belief, it is not necessary for a woman to have an orgasm for conception to take place. However, an unfulfilled, unsatisfactory sex life may well create marital stress and tension, which, as explained earlier, often appears to inhibit fertility. Furthermore, it is not always necessary for the semen to be deposited at the cervix, and many accidental pregnancies have resulted from the emission of semen at the entrance of the vagina (vulva). In general, however, the vaginal environment is hostile towards spermatozoa, being too acid for their prolonged survival (they are happiest in a slightly alkaline medium). Consequently, it is far better that the semen is deposited at the cervix as this reduces both the exposure of the spermatozoa to the acid vaginal secretions and the distance they have to travel before entering the uterus.

The importance of depositing the semen high in the vagina leads us on to what is probably the most common 'technical failure' during sex—premature ejaculation. In this condition sexual excitement on the part of the man is so intense that ejaculation takes place before the penis is sufficiently deep inside the vagina to ensure good deposition of semen at the cervix. (This condition is not to be confused with impotence, which is an inability of the man to produce and maintain an erection.) Premature ejaculation does not always lead to infertility by any means, and it is remarkable how spermatozoa can sometimes find their way along the length of the vagina to the uterus after having been deposited completely outside the vagina. Premature ejaculation may simply be due to inexperience, but can occur in response to emotional stress or conflict between partners, and men who suffer from this problem may benefit greatly from the advice and care of a sex therapist—sometimes called 'psychosexual counselling'. The woman can be taught ways to assist the man with this problem which, together with her sympathy and understanding, very often contribute greatly to its solution.

Premature ejaculation

One treatment frequently recommended begins with a period of complete abstinence from sex; this is followed by periods of early sexual contact between the partners, leading gradually to more intimate sexual practices, with intercourse finally taking place after several months of controlled build-up, which hopefully will eliminate the problem of excessive excitement which prevents penetration of the woman. A 'squeeze' technique is often employed to delay orgasm; the penis is squeezed firmly just before the point of orgasm and the sensation passes, allowing a further period before ejaculation. After a while entry of the penis into the vagina can be achieved. The man is often advised to spend time stimulating his partner's clitoris, in the hope of producing a simultaneous orgasm.

Impotence

Men who are impotent do not usually wait for infertility investigations before seeking help from doctors. The causes of male impotence are legion. They include physical injury, damage to the special nerves which cause erection (either by injury or disease), extreme old age, and certain drug therapies. However, in a very large proportion of impotent men the condition is the result of mental and emotional disturbances. A small proportion of men with physical causes may respond to treatment: for example, if impotence is a side effect of drug therapy, withdrawal of the drug will cure the condition. However, the majority of physical causes are incurable: many of the patients have serious diseases of the nervous system, or severe paralyses, often as the result of road accidents.

Men whose impotence is due to severe psychological problems need skilled assistance from psychiatrists and psychotherapists, but the outlook is usually good once the emotional and mental barriers have been breeched. Impotence can also be a transient and less serious problem; many men experience occasional periods of psychologically induced impotence. These often occur during bouts of severe depression and at times of emotional self-assessment and readjustment, which have been described by some as the 'male menopause'. As with premature ejaculation, impotence sometimes appears to be caused by emotional stress between the partners, and in such cases the sympathetic understanding of the woman, perhaps together with the help of a sex therapist, may be all that is necessary.

For those with true longstanding and incurable physical impotence several devices (prostheses) to produce an erection have recently become available. In the past, mechanical aids to erection have involved the surgical insertion of a plastic implant into the penis. This replaces the function of the normal 'rod of blood' which causes erection, but has the disadvantage that the penis is maintained in a semi-erect position for most of the time. A more recent invention consists of a pair of inflatable implants, a reservoir of fluid and a small pump mechanism placed in the scrotum. Prior to intercourse it is possible to pump fluid from the reservoir and inflate the device within the penis, and subsequently a valve can be released to allow the 'erection' to subside. This has the obvious advantage of allowing the patient to dress normally, but the device is much more expensive and the operation to fit it more difficult.

As far as fertility is concerned, the big question is whether these devices allow a man to achieve ejaculation and thus father a child. The answer is that it depends on the condition of the appropriate part of the nervous system. Erection is controlled by a chain of nerves in the parasympathetic nervous system, while ejaculation occurs by the action of nerves in the separate sympathetic nervous system. The sympathetic system gets the body ready for 'flight, fright and fight'—the blood is diverted from the stomach to the muscles of the legs and arms, the pupils of the eyes dilate, the heart and lungs speed up and sweating occurs. The parasympathetic system causes virtually the reverse actions. Thus, even if erection is impaired it may still be possible for the man to ejaculate providing that the relevant part of the nervous system is intact. Young men who are impotent following an injury, for example, may well be able to ejaculate with such a device in place. However, powerful psychological forces arising from the malfunction or disease may inhibit ejaculation even when prostheses are used and the nervous system is intact.

Painful intercourse

Sometimes infrequent intercourse, and a consequent delay in conceiving, is caused by reluctance on the part of the female partner. Worried by this, and perhaps not knowing to whom she should turn for advice, such a woman may well find herself consulting her doctor for infertility. When the doctor asks, 'how many times do you have intercourse each week?' the reply 'not many' is usually accompanied by an explanation of why. The reason why a woman does not enjoy sex is often pain or fear or both. An inability to relax the vaginal muscles (vaginal spasm, or vaginismus) can prevent penetration by the man, turning the sex act into an ordeal at best and a fiasco at worst. Intercourse can become a distressing fight rather than an expression of mutual love: this is obviously not at all conducive to fertility.

Many women who have psychological barriers to intercourse may find it difficult to admit to their partners, their doctors, and even to themselves that their problem is one of mental conditioning, and they often complain of pain during intercourse as an expression of their fears and misgivings. A doctor who, after examining the woman, can find no obvious cause for pain during intercourse may therefore ask tactful questions to seek a psychological cause. The outlook for the majority of women with problems of this nature is extremely good—nearly everyone builds up considerable prejudices and fears based on parental attitudes, schooltime myths, and early sexual encounters, but these are soon lost in the light of better information and experience.

Women who have such problems need careful counselling to help overcome their fear. The use of vaginal dilators (plastic devices shaped like a penis) is frequently very helpful. Dilators of increasing size are used over a period of time to achieve complete relaxation of the vaginal muscles. Occasionally the doctor will discover that the hymen (maidenhead) is still intact. The hymen is a thin membrane which in girls partially or completely covers the entrance to the vagina, and is normally broken when a woman first has sexual intercourse or often before, especially if tampons have been used during menstruation. If the hymen is unusually rigid, however, it may prevent entry of the penis. Similarly, the doctor may find an unusually small vaginal entrance. The hymen can easily be removed by a small operation and minor plastic surgery can open up the vaginal entrance.

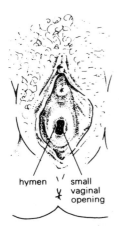

hymen   small vaginal opening

Position of the hymen. A hymen that is intact or a small vaginal opening may be the cause of difficulties with sexual intercourse.

Vaginal spasm may be the result of a 'strict' upbringing and indicate inhibition towards sex, even within marriage. Support, reassurance and advice and the patient understanding of the male partner are essential. Sometimes a good meal, a bottle of wine, soft lights and music can induce the necessary relaxation!

It is also possible that other causes of painful intercourse such as external or internal infections may delay conception, but in most cases these will be dealt with before help is sought for infertility. One other condition is worthy of mention here, however, since it can not only cause pain during intercourse, but also be a cause of infertility itself, by preventing ovulation. This condition is called endometriosis (see pp. 74–76 and 89).

2

Preliminary investigations

At the first consultation with the couple the investigating doctor will be looking initially for any possible clue which might point to the cause of the conception problem. Much can be gleaned by a few minutes of sensible questioning and the woman should not feel embarrassed or resentful at being asked a great number of questions, the immediate relevance of which may not always be apparent. As in all investigations much time-wasting effort and inconvenience can be caused by missing an important piece of information that could have been produced during the routine questioning at the beginning.

During my undergraduate days a fellow medical student was 'presenting' a woman complaining of infertility to our gynaecology chief and his students. We heard how her periods had stopped eight months previously, how she had menstruated regularly before that, and the student told us all about her past medical and social history. When he had finished the chief shook his head. 'Ask her something else,' he said, 'ask her what her weight has been doing.' My colleague went off, slightly ashamed at the omission of what might appear only a trivial point to most. He returned quickly to tell us that yes, she had been on a diet last year, and yes, she had lost two stone, and yes, her periods did stop just after the fall in weight, and there probably lay the answer. This demonstrates the importance of asking the right questions early on: if this

Routine questions for the woman

point had been overlooked, many unnecessary investigations might have been carried out. The experienced doctor will quickly assess the answers the woman gives and home in on those pieces of information which appear to be most relevant. Early on he or she would establish that there really is a problem—that a reasonable time has elapsed in trying for a pregnancy, that intercourse is satisfactory, takes place at approximately the right time during the menstrual cycle, and that there are no immediate problems that can be corrected or misconceptions (no pun intended) that can be elucidated.

Family and medical history

Infertility cannot be said to be inherited! However, family history can be significant, and it may be relevant to know, for instance, that several close relatives of the patient suffer from diabetes, or that one of her parents died of tuberculosis. More important, though, is the woman's previous medical history, and she will be expected to relate all the medical problems she may have had in the past. Serious illnesses, venereal diseases and operations may all be relevant. For instance, in the venereal disease gonorrhoea, infection may spread to the Fallopian tubes and cause blockage or damage to their delicate linings, severely limiting the chance of an ovum passing down them. Operations in the area of the pelvis, such as appendicectomy, may cause infections or the formation of scar tissue (adhesions) around the tubes and ovaries—with the same possible deleterious effects. I hasten to add that I am not implying that all women who have had their appendix removed are necessarily sterile; what I am saying is that it is a factor that the doctor will bear in mind during the course of later investigations, when it may be of some relevance.

Any operations on the gynaecological organs—uterus, Fallopian tubes, ovaries, vagina, vulva—must be recorded. Some patients are fairly ignorant of their own bodies and are not too sure about the various 'bits and pieces' of their reproductive apparatus. If such women have had an operation 'down there' they are frequently unsure of the details. Some are hampered by vocabulary and may be embarrassed to describe their symptons and ideas about the operation. However, the doctor can always check the records of the hospital concerned to find out the exact surgical details of what took place. A typical case might be a woman who has had an operation to remove an ectopic pregnancy (where the embryo starts to develop outside the uterus, most frequently in a Fallopian tube); in the days of upset, discomfort and anxiety that followed she may have become confused as to whether the surgeon had removed part of the Fallopian tube, or the whole tube, or the tube and the ovary—even though this was explained at the time.

The age at which a woman's periods first started (the menarche) is recorded. Most girls start to menstruate between 11 and 14, although variation on either side is quite common. The first few periods tend to be painless and ovulation does not take place; when ova are produced with each cycle then the periods tend to produce cramping and even pain to a greater or lesser degree. The age of the menarche is getting earlier and earlier in well-nourished societies and the menopause (when periods stop) later and later—thus the span of a women's fertility is gradually being extended. In underdeveloped countries this span is reduced and the menarche comes later. In Shakespeare's time the onset of a girl's periods occurred much later than it does in the healthier and better nourished days of this century: nowadays in Western countries 95 per cent of girls with normal ovarian functions will have menstruated by the age of 16. **Menstrual history**

A delay in the onset of periods may indicate that the ovaries are not functioning correctly. A complete absence of pain with periods and an irregular menstrual cycle may also suggest a failure or impairment of ovulation. The doctor will, of course, take a detailed menstrual history. Amenorrhoea (no menstrual bleeding at all for months, or even years) may also suggest that the ovaries are not functioning properly or that there is some deficiency in the chain of hormones which activate the menstrual cycle.

The same goes for scanty or irregular periods. It should be said straight away that sudden changes of surroundings or occupation, excessive worry, tension caused by exams, and marked weight loss may all cause temporary amenorrhoea which frequently ceases when surroundings, activities or weight return to normal. The classic cases of this are girls who go away to college or to work abroad. When periods stop, fear that they might be pregnant suddenly adds to their worries. However, women in this situation are not likely to come along to their doctor complaining of infertility; on the contrary, they are usually relieved to find out they are not pregnant right in the middle of their first term at college!

Women who suffer a marked drop in weight and cease to menstruate, however, frequently do seek medical help because they have not been able to conceive; usually they are 'discovered' at the first interview by a sensible doctor, as we saw at the beginning of the chapter. Going on to a weight-gaining diet is usually all that is required for periods to resume. We don't know the exact mechanism by which periods stop when weight drops, but periods, fertility, and nutrition are all closely interrelated. A very restrictive diet may reduce the woman's body weight to what it was before the menarche, or to a level at which she would not have the reserves of strength to support a pregnancy, and so it is understandable that the ovaries are 'switched off'. This is an oversimplification of the situation but it will have to suffice: the apparatus by which weight-related amenorrhoea (not to mention the effects of emotions and instinctive drives such as hate, rage, love, and hunger) is mediated lies in the hypothalamus—an area at the base of the brain just above the pituitary gland (see p. 31). Physiologists have much to discover about how this small but immensely important part of our brain works.

The effect of contraceptives

Another factor to be considered at the first visit is the method of contraception the couple have been using in the past (if any). The barrier methods, such as the sheath (condom) or diaphragm (Dutch cap) are not likely to have any effect on fertility after their use is stopped. The two other principal methods of contraception—oral contraceptives ('the pill') and the intrauterine device (IUCD, or coil)—can cause occasional problems.

Women who use oral contraceptives are often worried that they may have difficulty in becoming pregnant when they want to have a child, especially if they have been taking the pill for a considerable time. Happily, most women who stop taking the pill do not have to wait very long before becoming pregnant, and when problems do occur (i.e., if a woman does not begin to ovulate again and have normal periods), effective medical treatment is available. The reason why women are anxious about the effects of the pill is usually that they are aware that, by taking oral contraceptives, they are interfering with the usual hormone levels in their bodies. While this is a very understandable fear, it might reassure people to know more about how the pill works; now that oral contraceptives have been in use for nearly 30 years, our knowledge about them is considerable. They prevent conception in a variety of ways.

The most common type of pill contains synthetic oestrogen and progestogen hormones, and its main action is to prevent ovulation—the release of eggs from the ovary. These synthetic hormones are very similar to natural sex hormones which fulfil many functions in the body and circulate in relatively high levels during pregnancy. The body responds to the presence of these extra hormones in the bloodstream exactly as if it were pregnant—by switching off the ovulation mechanism. The pituitary gland stops producing hormones necessary to stimulate the ovary to release an egg. The mucus around the cervix becomes thicker and more hostile to spermatozoa. Again, this is similar to what happens in pregnancy, and so a woman taking the pill can be thought of as 'a little bit pregnant' hormonally speaking. As soon as the pill is not taken, the hormone levels fall and a 'withdrawal' bleed occurs; when the pill is taken cyclically for three weeks out of every four, a normal menstrual period is simulated with a withdrawal bleed occurring in the fourth week. If before starting the pill a woman was ovulating normally and experienced regular satisfactory periods it is likely that her normal periods will return immediately she stops taking the pill, particularly if she has been taking one of the modern low-dose preparations. A small number of women will experience 'post-pill amenorrhoea'; in these cases periods are usually switched on with one of the fertility drugs—more of this later.

Today this problem occurs much less frequently than a few years ago. In the early days, oral contraceptives were used by some practitioners to 'regularize' very irregular periods in certain women. We now know that these women were probably not ovulating regularly, or at all, and in some such cases the injudicious use of oral contraceptives may have had the effect of suppressing ovulation and the menstrual cycle after the pill is discontinued. Of course, the withdrawal bleed produced when taking oral contraceptives does appear to 'regularize' periods. But nowadays a doctor will not prescribe the pill unless satisfied that the woman's menstrual cycles have been normal and regular, suggesting normal ovulation, for at least a year. If not he or she would suggest some other form of contraception which does not run the risk of suppressing an already scanty pattern of ovulation.

Fertility and the IUCD The effect of the intrauterine contraceptive device (IUD or IUCD, usually simply referred to as 'the coil') on subsequent fertility is a frequently raised question to which, again, there are no clear-cut answers. There have been recent suggestions that IUCDs fitted to women who have not had a child may set up a low-grade inflammation in the lining of the womb (endometrium) which may not cause any symptoms of pain or fever, but which could delay subsequent fertility when the IUCD is removed. This is not a widespread problem since most women who have not had a child tend to want 100 per cent contraceptive protection and usually opt for the pill, since there is a small failure rate with an IUCD. However, some women who have not had a child, and who for medical or personal reasons cannot or will not take the pill regularly, are fitted with an IUCD. They do not usually have any problems in conceiving when it is taken out. Providing that the modern type of IUCD now in use is fitted properly and checked by a doctor experienced in family planning, the risk to subsequent fertility is minimal. Because of concern about the type of low-grade inflammation just mentioned, however, some practitioners would not recommend use of an IUCD by a childless woman unless extensive discussion had taken place. Women who have had previous episodes of pelvic inflammatory disease that were inadequately treated might experience a 'flare-up' when an IUCD is fitted, but the doctor will usually have excluded this possibility before offering to fit the device.

Quite a few patients seeking help for infertility will have been pregnant in the past. Gynaecology textbooks for doctors make a great distinction between the causes of infertility in a woman who has not conceived before (primary infertility) and the woman who has (secondary infertility). Obviously, the woman who has had a child (or even a pregnancy which ended in miscarriage) has demonstrated that she has, or at least has had, the ability to produce children—whereas this is not the case in women with primary infertility. Of course, the doctor will record full details of any previous pregnancies and, significantly, who fathered them. A woman whose second marriage is barren after she had children easily by her first husband, for instance, is bound to suspect that her second husband is infertile, but this is not always the case; the wise doctor will be slow to jump to any conclusions without proper investigations.

Previous pregnancies or miscarriages

Details of deliveries of children in the past are important. Infections after childbirth may in a few unfortunate women result in subsequent infertility, for example, if the lining of the Fallopian tube was destroyed. Any findings reported by the surgeon at a Caesarean section may also be relevant. Any problems, such as infection, following a Caesarean operation will also be considered.

In many cases, of course, pregnancies may have occurred in the past but not reached full term; the occurrence of a miscarriage may be encouraging in that it indicates that the apparatus for conception is functioning to some extent at least. The typical 'Hollywood miscarriage', as portrayed in films or popular fiction, in which the woman has a miscarriage and then is unable to conceive ever again, is in fact extremely rare. Miscarriage is a much more common event than people realize: one in five pregnancies ends in miscarriage. Often miscarriage is a form of quality control whereby the body can 'discard' a substandard fetus. A quick clean miscarriage with no problems afterwards will not cause sterility. But infection of the uterus or Fallopian tubes following a miscarriage can cause infertility in some cases.

This raises the ugly question of illegal or 'backstreet' abortions in which a woman is induced to miscarry by the introduction of an instrument into the uterus, disturbing the fetus. If the procedure is not performed in clean and sterile conditions, an infection can be set up, which in some cases might damage the reproductive organs. Even legal abortions—terminations of pregnancy—performed in approved hospitals and clinics are occasionally followed by infection and/or damage to the uterus or Fallopian tubes. However, since the woman is under competent medical surveillance, these complications are usually treated swiftly and the chances of subsequent infertility are therefore considerably reduced. I should mention that doctors do not often use the term miscarriage—they call a miscarriage a 'spontaneous abortion', and what we all know as an 'abortion' they call a 'therapeutic abortion' or 'termination of pregnancy'. I shall discuss the subject of miscarriage, its possible causes and ways of preventing it in greater detail on pp. 92 to 101.

Breast feeding

Nature, of course, produces its own period of infertility after the birth of a baby. During breast feeding most women do not menstruate and are unlikely to become pregnant. About one-third of women will ovulate *before* weaning is completed and are therefore fertile, and most doctors therefore advocate the use of contraceptives during breast feeding unless a pregnancy is wanted. However, anyone seeking advice for infertility following childbirth should be aware that it is normal for breast feeding to prevent ovulation and therefore conception.

The physical examination

It is usual for the doctor to examine the woman after taking the medical history. With the advent of complex biochemical tests that can be performed in the laboratory and the increasing use of medical technology, especially ultrasound scanning, the importance of the physical examination by the doctor is declining in infertility work, as it is to some extent in almost all fields of medicine. Nowadays the cause of most cases of infertility in women could be discovered with a few blood tests and a laparoscopy (more of this later) without the classic medical exam. However, where the cause of the infertility is one of the more obscure varieties, a clue may be obtained from a doctor's examination which will put the line of blood tests, x-rays etc., on the right track and occasionally cut out unnecessary procedures and investigations. For this reason it is important that each woman should be carefully examined at the beginning of infertility investigations.

The examination can be divided into two parts—a general examination of the woman's whole body, and the internal pelvic examination, which specifically allows the doctor to feel the state of the reproductive organs with his or her hands. Any suspicion produced by the medical history that the infertility might be a result of a generalized disease, such as an abnormality of the thyroid gland, will guide the doctor in the brief examination of the head, chest, abdomen and legs to a more thorough examination of the area under suspicion—in this case the thyroid gland.

The general examination

An overall impression of the woman's weight-to-height ratio is noted—is she unusually thin or overweight?—and her development both physically and sexually. We have already seen that body weight can have an effect on periods. Very occasionally, a woman who is severely underweight will deny that she has been dieting or has lost a lot of weight; a possible explanation is the condition of anorexia nervosa, where dieting or refusing to eat becomes an obsession. Periods cease when weight falls, which, some doctors believe, is the subconscious intention of a woman with this condition.

A short, stunted physique might suggest a rare chromosomal abnormality, such as Turner's syndrome, in which the woman has only one X sex chromosome instead of the normal double X combinations; such women are infertile but the condition is very uncommon. However, serious chromosomal problems of this nature are usually diagnosed long before infertility becomes a problem. In cases where menstruation has been absent, infrequent, or scanty, the doctor will look for the absence of secondary sexual characteristics—breast development, normal female body curvature, feminine hair distribution, etc.—which might suggest a deficiency of female sex hormones. More masculine characteristics, such as heavy facial hair growth, moderate or severe acne, a receding hairline, and lack of breast enlargement and hip curvature, might also indicate a deficiency of female sex hormones or an increase in the usually small quantity of male hormones which are produced by the adrenal glands and are always present in a woman's body. In extremely rare cases masculine characteristics might be due to an ovarian tumour called an arrhenoblastoma, which secretes male hormones. These are, however, very uncommon. Facial hair in women to a greater or lesser extent is, by contrast, quite common—but in the majority of women there is no underlying hormonal imbalance at all.

The thyroid gland is usually felt with the fingertips, and 'palpated'. The thyroid lies in the neck, just in front of the windpipe, and is shield-like in appearance (which is what the word 'thyroid' means). It controls the general level of metabolism, the rate at which the body 'ticks over'. Increased activity of the thyroid gland speeds up the pulse rate, makes a person feel warm even when others feel cold, burns up a good deal of extra energy—and tends to shorten or abolish menstrual periods. Decreased activity of the thyroid slows the body down in several ways, and may prolong menstrual periods and make them heavy (menorrhagia). Both states may affect fertility. Such malfunction of the thyroid may sometimes be felt by the doctor as an enlargement of the whole gland or one of its lobes.

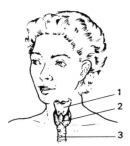

Position of the thyroid gland.
1 Larynx 2 Thyroid gland
3 Windpipe (trachea)

In a few instances, infertility may be due to abnormalities in the brain. A small tumour in the pituitary gland in the base of the brain can interfere with normal hormone production and might occasionally account for infertility in an otherwise healthy woman. Such a tumour could lead to suppression of the periods and a discharge from the breasts (galactorrhoea). It could also cause the pituitary gland to enlarge and press on the nerves leading from the retina at the back of the eyes to the brain. This can cause changes in the area where the nerves reach the back of the eye which are sometimes visible on inspecting the retina with an ophthalmoscope, and may also impair the lateral field of vision. Although this is relatively uncommon I thought I would mention it as some women might be puzzled as to why the doctor should spend a minute or two looking into her eyes with a small lighted instrument, or testing her eyesight and visual fields.

In these days of good nourishment and high standards of hygiene, tuberculosis (TB) is not nearly so common as half a century ago. Listening to the chest for signs of pulmonary TB is normally unrewarding, but a chest x-ray may occasionally be requested to exclude this and other chest problems routinely. TB can spread from other sites in the body to infect the Fallopian tubes. This is a well-recognized cause of infertility, but is now very uncommon in Western countries.

The blood pressure is checked routinely. The abdomen is examined briefly: any operation scars are noted, especially those made to remove the appendix, an ectopic pregnancy or an ovarian cyst, since during the taking of the medical history these operations may well have been forgotten in the heat of the moment. It is not uncommon at all for a doctor to ask, 'Any serious operations in the past?' and receive the reply 'No,' only to find an appendicectomy scar! 'Oh, but that wasn't a serious operation, doctor' says the patient. The doctor might well be justified in replying, 'Well, not in your case, as it turned out.' In fact some people die each year from such 'simple' operations as removing the appendix or an ectopic pregnancy. *Any* operation in the pelvic or lower abdominal area is relevant to the investigation of infer-

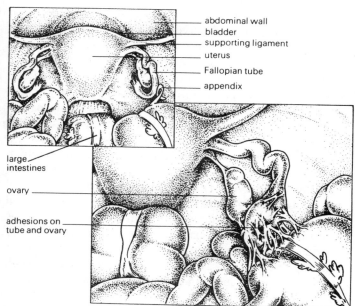

abdominal wall
bladder
supporting ligament
uterus
Fallopian tube
appendix

large intestines

ovary

adhesions on tube and ovary

Left: A normal uterus and ovary (inset), and one bound down with adhesions, both seen from the rear. An abdominal operation such as removal of the appendix can cause adhesions (scar tissue) which may affect fertility.

tility, so before you go in to see the doctor it might be a good idea to make a list of the medical problems you have had in the past, with dates and places of treatment, and any medical problems in your immediate family, so that you can produce a complete list when asked.

The internal pelvic examination

Last of all comes the internal pelvic examination. Unfortunately, the thought of this fills some women with anxiety and apprehension, especially if they have not been examined before. Sometimes this anxiety tends to cloud the medical history-taking and preliminary chat with the doctor, and several important questions might not be fully taken in because the woman is working herself into a state about the pelvic examination. It is rather like sitting in the dentist's waiting room and being unable to concentrate on what one is reading—which is why, I presume, glossy picture magazines are provided rather than books by Jacob Bronowski. Some women may have also been primed by friends who have exaggerated beyond reason the 'torture' of a pelvic examination.

Let me say at the outset that the internal pelvic examination should be nothing worse than uncomfortable; in the majority of cases it is completely painless. Occasionally, there might be slight pain when, for example, the doctor discovers that there is tenderness of the ovaries and Fallopian tubes and then tries further to assess the degree of tenderness; but in the normal healthy female a pelvic examination conducted in a relaxed and professional atmosphere should not hurt at all. Any doctor who does hurt a woman during a routine examination should be rebuked by the patient in no uncertain terms. It is true, I regret to say, that a very few gynaecologists and other practitioners seem to feel that an examination which does not hurt to some extent is probably not thorough enough, while a very few are simply uncaring, hamfisted and boorish. I might add that a few women doctors as well as men are included in this, thankfully small, group. A rigorous, painful examination is likely to undermine any confidence and trust between the patient and the doctor carrying out the investigations. Any aggressive types such as those described should be avoided and another opinion sought.

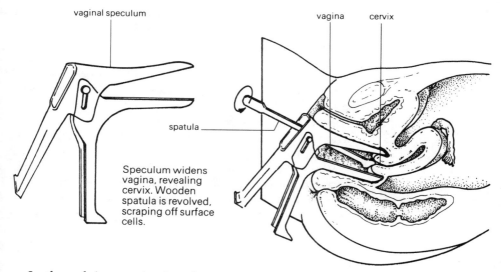

vaginal speculum

vagina   cervix

spatula

Speculum widens
vagina, revealing
cervix. Wooden
spatula is revolved,
scraping off surface
cells.

In the pelvic examination the organs are felt through the layers of skin, fat and muscle, and minor abnormalities can be difficult to detect. Of much more use are the techniques of direct vision allowed by the laparoscope, which require a stay in hospital and the use of a general anaesthetic (this comes much later in the investigations: see p. 83). But the value of the pelvic examination lies in the fact that gross problems, such as active pelvic inflammatory disease or major abnormalities of the reproductive organs, can be detected (or at least ruled out) as early as possible.

How a cervical smear is taken for testing.

If the woman has not had a cervical smear test (sometimes called a 'Pap' smear after the doctor who pioneered it, George Papanicolaou) within the previous year or so, the doctor will perform one at this stage. The test is designed to detect 'premalignant' changes in the cells of the cervix (neck of the womb), which are an early warning signal of developing cancer. If necessary, treatment to prevent a cancer developing can be initiated immediately. It is a very easy test to do, and although it does not have much to do with infertility directly, the opportunity to perform it can be thought of as a bonus. The woman lies on her back or side and a bivalved speculum is inserted gently into the vagina. By closing the handles the two 'valves' are opened, allowing a good view of the cervix. Using a small wooden spatula a layer of cells is gently scraped from the surface of the cervix, particularly from the likely danger area just inside the opening (cervical os). Only moderate pressure is required and the procedure is without pain. The scraping of cells is spread out (smeared) on to a glass microscope slide and the cells 'fixed' by dipping or spraying them in an alcohol preservative. The slide is then sent to a trained cytologist, who will inspect the cells under the microscope and make a report (this usually takes a few days to come back).

While the speculum is in position for the smear, the doctor will have a good look at the state of the cervix and the part of the vagina visible. Particular note will be taken of any vaginal discharge, which might benefit from treatment, but is probably not a cause of infertility. More important is the state of the cervix itself. Reduced fertility can sometimes be due to chronic infections of the cervix (cervicitis), since this produces a hostile environment which is usually too acid for the spermatozoa and perhaps does not allow the essential changes known as capacitation to take place. Incidentally, when doctors say 'chronic' they mean 'longstanding', and when they say 'acute' they mean 'of quick onset' or 'of short duration'. The terms relate to time only and not to severity. It is wrong to say 'the pain was very acute'—an acute pain is one which comes on quickly.

While viewing the cervix the doctor will note the amount and quality of the cervical mucus present. Simple tests and a microscope examination of a sample of the cervical mucus may also give hints about whether or not ovulation is occurring, but these rather old-fashioned methods have been superseded by more accurate ones.

Occasionally doctors perform a test called endometrial biopsy, which consists of removing a small piece of tissue from the endometrium, or lining of the uterus. In the second half of the menstrual cycle, after ovulation has occurred, the appearance of the endometrium changes; it becomes markedly glandular ('secretory') whereas before ovulation its appearance is 'proliferative'. By introducing a small grooved rod with a relatively sharp end into the womb through the cervical canal a small sample of the endometrium (a biopsy) can be scraped out and sent for

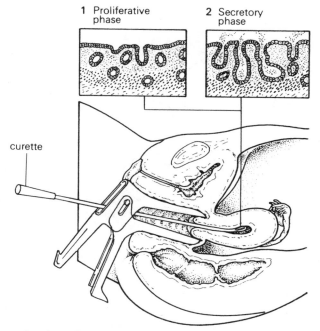

1 Proliferative phase

2 Secretory phase

curette

Performing an endometrial biopsy. A small sample of cells from the lining of the womb is scraped off during the second half of the menstrual cycle (secretory phase). This can indicate whether ovulation is occurring.

examination. Its appearance under the microscope helps determine whether ovulation is occurring and whether the uterine lining has become receptive, to allow implantation and growth of the fertilized egg. This procedure can be painful to a varying degree.

Having taken the smear and looked at the cervix the doctor will perform the bimanual internal pelvic examination. Usually the woman lies on her back with her knees flopped apart, or with her heels together and knees bent at right angles. The doctor, wearing a lubricated glove, inserts first and second fingers into the vagina while the other hand palpates (feels) the lower abdomen. In a few women the vaginal muscles tense up (vaginismus) and the doctor will patiently wait until the woman can relax completely before continuing.

The fingers will rest against the cervix, and the uterus will be felt against the fingers in the vagina and the hand on the abdomen. An estimate of its size and shape can be made in all but exceptionally fat women. A knobbly uneven uterus would suggest the presence of benign swellings of the muscle known as fibroids. A normal

The technique of bimanual examination. The doctor can feel the size and shape of the uterus, and its mobility.

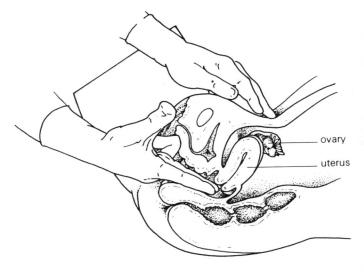

ovary

uterus

womb has a fair degree of mobility, and where the womb is found to be fixed, there is a strong possibility that the woman has had previous episodes of pelvic inflammatory disease—and this infection may have caused blocked Fallopian tubes. A tender, relatively immobile womb might also be due to the condition of endometriosis, which can also cause infertility (see pp. 74–76).

A womb which is badly misshapen by multiple fibroids may not allow satisfactory implantation of the fertilized ovum, and even if this does take place, miscarriage early in the pregnancy may result. The finding of one or two small fibroids (most women over 30 years of age have one or more fibroids, usually very small indeed) is hardly likely to account for infertility. A tiny shrunken womb might suggest that there is some maldevelopment of the reproductive organs.

The ovaries, which are about the size and shape of large almonds, will also be felt. Do not forget that the Fallopian tubes are only about three inches long, so the ovaries lie quite close to the uterus—because of badly drawn diagrams in some books, many women think the ovaries sit high up in the abdomen! In fact they are situated well down in the pelvis at the ends of the Fallopian tubes, so that when an ovum is released on to the ovary surface the fimbriae (fronds) of the tubes are right there ready to pick the ovum up. If the ovaries are felt to be enlarged, they may be 'polycystic'—containing numerous small cysts. (This condition, which may be part of the Stein-Leventhal syndrome, is discussed on p. 88). Thickening of the tubes and ovaries often suggests that there has been inflammation (pelvic inflammatory disease) in the past, or, if the tubes and ovaries are tender, that inflammation is more recent or current. In both cases the result may be blockage of the Fallopian tubes.

Any signs of these abnormalities of the uterus or ovaries will be investigated by more specialized tests (see pp. 79–82 and pp. 88–89), and appropriate treatment offered as necessary. In the next chapter, however, we shall look at some simple tests that are a routine part of most infertility investigations, and we shall consider how the doctor plans the sequence of further tests and procedures.

3

Simple tests

The way a doctor plans the course of the investigations is open to much variation. One important factor is the woman's age. For example, if a woman aged 38 wishes for infertility investigations and treatment (which could take up to two years) the doctor must get moving quickly and not waste time. A younger woman who has only tried for a baby for about a year, and who from her history and examination does not appear to have any serious problem, might have her investigations in a more leisurely fashion. Another factor which will help to determine the type and sequence of tests is the medical history. A woman who has not menstruated for a year or two will require different management to a woman who has no suggestion of menstrual irregularity and whose problem might be blocked Fallopian tubes. However, all things being equal, most doctors start off by asking the woman to keep temperature charts and recommend that the man has a seminalysis or sperm test at this stage.

Both of these are important. Temperature charts offer an easy method of trying to see if ovulation is occurring: this must be established early on, since about 20 per cent of cases of female infertility are due to ovulatory failure. In addition, because filling in the charts involves a sustained effort on the part of the woman, they give an indication of her motivation. If she cannot be bothered to keep temperature charts, just how keen is she to conceive? Does she attend the clinic because her husband has sent her, or do both partners genuinely want to proceed with investigations?

The seminalysis, where the man collects a sample of seminal fluid for examination, is equally important, because the results can determine which partner should be investigated first. There is not much point in proceeding to perform all kinds of tests, and even some surgical procedures, on the woman if the seminalysis shows that the man is almost certainly infertile. The correct specimen containers and instructions are often provided at this first visit. I shall look further into the question of when the man should be investigated in the next chapter.

Temperature charts

If you are given temperature charts, you will be asked to fill them in every day for at least a month and probably for three or four months. A typical printed chart is shown overleaf. You will be asked to take your temperature (and you may need instruction on this from the nurse) daily and record it on the chart. It is important to do this as soon as you wake up each morning, that is to say, before you raise the temperature artificially by smoking or drinking tea or coffee, or lower it artificially by cleaning your teeth with cold water. As you can see from the illustration, in the first half of the cycle the temperature is slightly lower than the second half after ovulation takes place. This is known as a 'biphasic' pattern. Typically, just before ovulation there is a little 'kick down' and then at ovulation there is a rise of nearly 0.5°C (1°F), which is sustained until menstruation takes place. If pregnancy occurs the woman will not menstruate (though she may bleed very lightly— 'implantation bleeding') and the temperature remains slightly elevated.

The charts are started on the first day of menstrual bleeding and a new chart commenced at the beginning of the next period. It is usual to ask the woman to mark on the card the days on which sexual intercourse took place.

If they have been kept properly, these charts are extremely useful and offer a great deal of information. At the next visit to the clinic they provide the answer to these questions:

1. Is the pattern biphasic (does it seem likely that the woman is ovulating)?
2. Are the menstrual periods prolonged, heavy, light, scanty, occasionally absent?

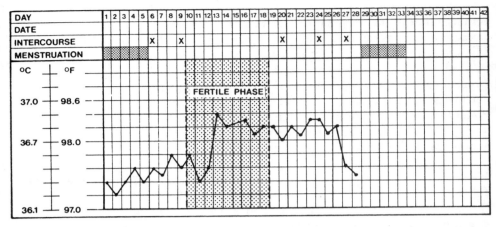

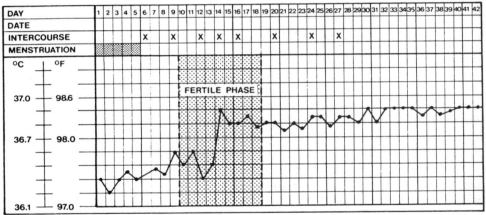

Typical temperature charts.
Top: Normal pattern for
ovulation. Above: Pattern for
ovulation and pregnancy,
with prolonged elevated
temperature. Little or no
elevation would indicate that
ovulation has not occurred.

3. When does ovulation appear to occur in relation to the periods? (Some women ovulate later than the 13th or 14th day if their cycle is longer than average.)

4. Most importantly, is intercourse occurring at the optimum time for conception, i.e., near to ovulation?

Now, unless the woman's medical history and examination suggest any abnormalities that require immediate investigation (such as a suspected pituitary gland tumour), many doctors will leave more complex texts to the second and subsequent visits, and see the woman (or the couple) again when the completed temperature charts and seminalysis results are available. Unless there is a really urgent need to get on with the more complex tests the doctor will take the initial investigations rather slowly and simply, because some couples will conceive early on in infertility investigations after they have been reassured by the doctor—sometimes after only one visit. So, don't be surprised if that is all that happens at your first visit—history-taking, examination, provision of temperature charts to fill in and a specimen container for seminalysis. Conversely, don't be alarmed if any further tests are ordered at this stage. Doctors vary in their approach, and some may do initial screening tests such as a chest x-ray, thyroid function tests, etc., as a matter of systematic routine rather than because they particularly suspect, say, some malfunction of the thyroid gland.

The postcoital test

Many doctors like to perform a 'postcoital test' early on, particularly at the second visit. The couple are asked to have sexual intercourse between two and four hours before their appointment with the doctor. The woman should not bathe, shower, or douche herself before going to the doctor's clinic, as this may wash the sperm away. The doctor will inspect the cervix with a vaginal speculum (the same type that is used to take a smear) and a small blob of cervical mucus is taken, placed upon a slide and examined there and then under a microscope. The test is painless. The doctor will look for the presence of spermatozoa, and, if they are present, whether they are moving about freely.

Finding no spermatozoa, along with a low sperm count at seminalysis, would suggest that the man might be infertile and should have further tests; the finding of many dead spermatozoa or vibrating spermatozoa, stuck within the mucus, might indicate the presence of antisperm antibodies (p. 63).

Sometimes there is an unusual explanation for the absence of spermatozoa at the postcoital test. On occasion I have met women who have practised vigorous vaginal washing (douching) immediately after intercourse; this does not allow time for the spermatozoa to penetrate the cervical mucus and get into the womb. At the postcoital test there was no sign of spermatozoa, not even a trace of semen, yet the results of seminalysis were good. One such woman had been brought up in a convent, where cleanliness was thought to be next to godliness, and she felt that the presence of semen inside her vagina, even for an hour or two, was in some way unclean, and following intercourse rushed off to the bathroom. I am happy to say that when she discontinued immediate vaginal douching she conceived after two months. This uncommon cause of infertility would not have come to light without the postcoital test—a safe, simple but extremely useful procedure. Its only problem is that it makes some men late for work on the morning of their wife's appointment, and it is sometimes a little embarrassing to explain why to their bosses!

4

Male infertility

A certain amount of strain and mistrust can easily arise in the relationship of a couple who fail to produce a much-wanted baby. It is important for both partners to face the prospect of infertility together and not to apportion blame—either consciously or subconsciously—to the other. It sometimes happens that men are reluctant to come forward for examination, even though they may accept that their wives may undergo a lengthy process of investigation. This reluctance may be because the man (mistakenly) associates fertility with virility, or sexual prowess, and is afraid—perhaps subconsciously—of being found to be infertile. However, it is very important that the male partner should have an examination of his semen performed as early as possible in the course of the infertility investigations. This is known as seminal analysis or seminalysis for short, and is also often referred to as a 'sperm count'. In a considerable proportion of couples who are investigated, a problem is found in the man (estimates vary between 10 and 50 per cent), and because of this, most doctors are reluctant to proceed with investigations on the female partner until a seminalysis has been performed.

In most cases, the result of the seminalysis will play an important part in determining what further tests (if any) should be carried out on both the man and the woman. For example, it might be found that the man is not producing spermatozoa at all (azoospermia). In this case there is obviously little point in proceeding with investigations on the woman. A man who is shown to be

When should the man be investigated?

azoospermic is usually referred to a urologist for specialist help. (A urologist is a surgeon who specializes in the diseases of the kidneys and bladders of both men and women, and problems associated with the male reproductive organs—prostate, seminal vesicles, vasa deferentia, testes and penis.) Unfortunately, however, there is very often nothing that can be done to help in such cases.

If the result of the seminalysis is very good, investigations on the woman should be continued. Should all these prove negative, i.e., if no apparent cause of infertility in the woman can be found, the man might then be sent for more specialized tests despite his seemingly normal sperm count. The results of these may also fail to reveal any cause of infertility in the man. Happily, however, in many cases where no reason for infertility can be detected in either partner, a pregnancy eventually ensues. This frequently happens shortly after completion of tests, presumably because the couple is reassured by the knowledge that nothing appears to be wrong.

Low sperm count

If the results of the seminalysis show a moderate to low sperm count, the man is often referred to a urologist for help. Further tests can be carried out, including at least two or three additional seminalyses to check whether the impairment is temporary or permanent. Usually, however, doctors will recommend that simple investigations also be carried out simultaneously on the woman for several reasons. Firstly, many men with low or moderately low sperm counts are fertile (i.e., they can father a child), and secondly, there may be some easily remedied cause of infertility in the woman. She may not be ovulating, for example, and this can often be rectified by using drugs to stimulate ovulation. From the practical point of view there is more chance of helping a subfertile woman than a subfertile man given the present state of our knowledge—as will be explained later.

On the whole, female infertility investigations are supervised by gynaecologists, whereas male infertility tests are conducted by urologists. Both are assisted by doctors in allied fields, such as endocrinologists (hormone specialists), and by laboratory and scientific personnel.

The majority of men undergoing further investigations, therefore, will be those whose sperm counts are low and whose partners have undergone simple investigations and have been found normal. In a large proportion of couples where the man attends a male clinic, a pregnancy will be achieved within six months—the figure has been shown to be over 50 per cent in two separate studies. This success rate may owe more to the reassurance imparted by the examinations than to the efficacy of treatment.

Although most descriptions of male fertility centre on the sperm count, this is by no means an infallible yardstick. It is just not possible to say with certainty that one man has a low sperm count and is therefore infertile, or that another has a high sperm count and is obviously fertile. There are many exceptions to both cases. I shall go into this in more detail in the section on seminalysis later in this chapter; but before doing so I would like to outline how spermatozoa, the male reproductive cells, are produced and function, and how they travel through the male sexual organs to the outside world.

Spermatozoa

Spermatozoa (or simply, sperm) are tiny tadpole-shaped cells; each has a long whiplike tail which permits it a considerable degree of mobility, and a head full of nuclear protein containing half the number of chromosomes required to construct a person. A female ovum (or egg

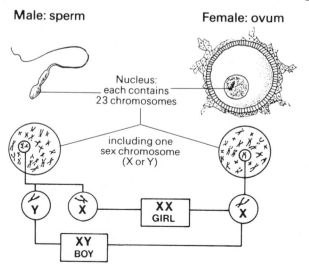

Male: sperm   Female: ovum

Nucleus: each contains 23 chromosomes

including one sex chromosome (X or Y)

Y   X   **XX GIRL**   X

XY BOY

Spermatazoa and ova each contain 23 chromosomes which join at fertilization to form the normal 46 chromosomes in every human cell. Chromosomes from the father always determine the sex of a child, as sperm may carry X or Y chromosomes, whereas an ovum only carries an X chromosome. An XY combination produces a boy, XX a girl.

cell) also contains half the number of chromosomes required, and when a spermatozoon penetrates an ovum their chromosomes fuse and they become a single cell— the fertilized ovum, which will eventually develop into a fetus. The spermatozoon will also carry the important X or Y sex chromosome which will determine whether the new person is female or male respectively. Spermatozoa are manufactured in the testes, beginning at puberty and continuing throughout a man's life into old age. The production of spermatozoa by the testes is stimulated by a hormone (follicle–stimulating hormone) emitted from the pituitary gland at the base of the brain.

Structure of the testes

Spermatazoa are produced in tubules of the testis and stored in the epididymis. Sperm travel up the vasa deferentia and mix with secretions from the seminal vesicles and prostate gland to form the ejaculate.

The testes each consist of a very long, thin tube wound tightly on itself, rather like the elastic inside a golfball; on top of the testes, which are the size of large walnuts, sits a slightly wider tube, again folded on itself, called the epididymis. Under the influence of hormones from the pituitary gland spermatozoa develop in the cells lining the tubes of the testes. When mature they are released into the bore of the tube and pass along to be stored in the

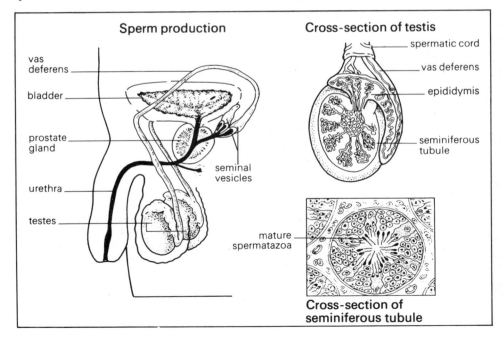

Sperm production

Cross-section of testis

vas deferens

bladder

prostate gland

urethra

testes

seminal vesicles

spermatic cord

vas deferens

epididymis

seminiferous tubule

mature spermatazoa

Cross-section of seminiferous tubule

epididymis. The epididymis is connected to the vas deferens—the long thickwalled muscular tube which sends the spermatozoa on their way to the outside world.

The spermatozoa are conducted by the vas deferens up into the abdominal cavity, along the base of the bladder, and through the prostate gland into the urethra, which will conduct them through the penis and out of the body. While passing under the base of the bladder the spermatozoa and the fluid surrounding them, together known as the ejaculate, are joined by a secretion from two glands known as the seminal vesicles. Another secretion, produced by the prostate gland, precedes the ejaculate in its journey from the prostate to the penis. This is known as the prostatic fluid and is alkaline in character. Among many other supposed functions, the prostatic fluid ensures that the path travelled by the spermatozoa through the urethra is at the right degree of alkalinity; it no doubt also removes any cell debris which may impede the path of the ejaculate.

Undescended testis

The two testes are originally formed early in fetal development in the abdomen, near the kidneys, and as the fetus develops they gradually move down, passing through a canal in the groin (the inguinal canal) so that at birth they are in the bag of skin known as the scrotum. It is thought that the testes are suspended outside the body in this fashion to permit them to function at a temperature several degrees lower than that of the rest of the body.

It is not uncommon for one or both of the testes to be arrested in their descent so that at birth they are still within the abdominal cavity—a condition known, naturally enough, as undescended testis. There are two reasons why an undescended testis should not be allowed to remain within the abdominal cavity. Firstly, intra-abdominal testes do not work properly and this may be a function of the higher body temperature that they are subjected to. More importantly, they have a significant tendency to develop malignant tumours. Testes which have become lodged in the groin canal can sometimes be brought down into the scrotum by a small operation, usually performed during early childhood, called an orchidopexy (the Greek term *orchid* being applied to anything pertaining to the testis). Intra–abdominal testes which cannot be brought down into the scrotum are usually removed in late childhood because of the cancer risk just mentioned. Unfortunately, it is not uncommon for a testis which has been successfully brought down by an operation to fail to produce spermatozoa. However, one functioning testis is generally sufficient to ensure fertility, and if the other was properly descended at birth or soon after, no problem usually arises.

The prostate gland

I must say a brief word about the prostate gland, because in addition to a great desire for people to call it 'the prostrate', few seem to understand its position within the male apparatus. As I have implied, scientists are still unsure of all the functions of the prostate gland and it is the subject of much research. The prostate gland is a walnut-sized organ which encircles the neck of the bladder, rather like a hand grasping the neck of a bottle. Through it passes the urethra—a small muscular tube which conducts urine from the bladder through the penis. At the prostate gland

The prostate gland surrounds the bladder neck. Enlargement causes difficulties in passing urine, and prolonged infections of the prostate can affect fertility.

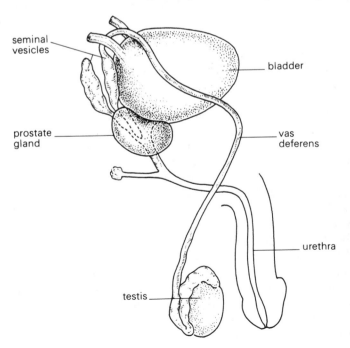

seminal vesicles

bladder

prostate gland

vas deferens

urethra

testis

the urethra is joined by the two vasa deferentia from the testes. Thus the male urethra is used not only for the passage of urine but for the passage of spermatozoa as well. As most people know, during old age the prostate gland tends to enlarge, narrowing the urethra and inhibiting the passage of urine. This condition frequently requires removal of the gland, or parts of it—an operation known as prostatectomy. Fertility can be impaired by long–term infections of the prostate. Men with such infections have sometimes been successful in making their partners pregnant after a course of suitable antibiotics.

In seminalysis, the man collects a sample of ejaculate in a container provided by the doctor. The sample should be collected directly, i.e., following masturbation. Interrupted intercourse may lead to an incomplete collection since the first portion of the ejaculate, which contains the majority of sperm, may be missed. Specimens collected in a contraceptive sheath (condom) are generally of no use, because most condoms are coated with a spermicidal compound which destroys the spermatozoa.

Seminalysis (the sperm count)

It is helpful if the man has abstained from masturbation and intercourse for two or three days prior to the collection in order to maximize the numbers of spermatozoa present. The sample must be delivered to the laboratory within two to four hours of collection, and sooner if possible. The specimen container is usually made of plastic, as this material produces less of a 'cold shock' to the spermatozoa than glass. The man is usually given a printed instruction sheet with it, which will request him to warm the container to body heat before ejaculation and to maintain it at this temperature for at least 15 minutes afterwards. Research has shown that if this is done and thereafter cooling is allowed to take place gradually, no extra warm wrapping is required during transportation to the laboratory.

In the laboratory the sample of semen is examined under the microscope. What are the doctors looking for? The quantity of the ejaculate usually varies between 2 and 6 ml, and it will be alkaline. The number of spermatozoa counted should be at least 20 million per ml of fluid, and preferably much higher; 40 per cent or more should be

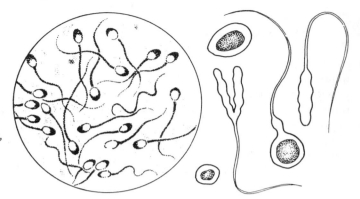

Right: Normal spermatazoa, as seen under a microscope. Far right: Examples of abnormal sperm, greatly enlarged.

actively motile (i.e., seen to be actively swimming by wriggling their bodies). A further search is made for abnormal cells and spermatozoa may be noticed with double heads, double tails or short tails. A normal sample should contain less than 30 per cent of these abnormal forms. The size of the individual cells is usually assessed, and although it does not matter if all the cells are large, or all are small, seminal fluid that contains sperm cells of different sizes may well be associated with subfertility. The levels of other substances in the semen may be relevant; for example, a large number of a certain type of white blood cell indicates a likelihood that the man has a prostate infection, which can impair fertility.

These criteria are the usual ones applied to the analysis of semen, but the results depend upon the circumstances in which the collection was made, and indeed upon various interpretations by the microscopist performing the analysis. A great many factors will influence the actual numbers and quality of the spermatozoa in each individual collection for seminalysis. Obviously, if intercourse has been extremely frequent, the count tends to be somewhat lowered as the spermatozoa are produced on demand. The sperm generation cycle can take between six and ten weeks. Counts may also depend on the physical condition of the man and indeed even on the time of day the collection was made. However, these are usually subtle variations in the results of the seminalysis rather than the gross abnormalities which are usually taken to indicate subfertility. If a man produces less than 20 million spermatozoa per ml he is considered to be 'oligospermic', and a man who produces no spermatozoa is termed 'azoospermic'. Should oligospermia or azoospermia be recorded initially, further collections are always obtained to check the result.

Seminalysis is open to a great deal of debate, and assessment of male fertility is still bedevilled by the impossibility of defining fertility purely in terms of the sperm count. For instance, the figure of 20 million sperms per ml has been widely regarded as an approximate dividing line between fertility and infertility, but even this figure is subject to doubt. As long ago as 1951 a very large study analysed the sperm counts of 1,000 fertile and 1,000 infertile couples. Of the infertile couples, 16 per cent of the husbands had sperm counts below 20 million per ml, compared with 5 per cent of the husbands of the fertile pairs. In other words, 84 per cent of the husbands of infertile marriages had sperm counts over 20 million per ml, but many men with counts of less than 20 million were fertile.

There is also some disagreement about what constitutes an abnormal form. In one study, photomicrographs of 500 sperms were sent to 47 experts and differing opinions on 50 per cent of the specimens were received. A man's spermatozoa may be abnormal because of a specific chromosome deficiency; this tends to be a permanent condition. Some abnormal forms may be due to environmental factors; this is not necessarily a permanent condition, but it is not easy to distinguish these two groups.

The man's medical history

As we have said, if repeated seminalysis shows persistently low sperm counts, the man may be referred for further investigations by a male infertility specialist. The first step will be to take a complete medical history. The investigating doctor will be looking out for any illnesses or conditions, past or present, which could possibly cause (or contribute to) infertility.

He or she may well begin by asking whether there was any problem in childhood with the descent of the testes into the scrotum and in particular whether any operations were performed in childhood. This is because, as I mentioned earlier, testes which have to be brought down by an operation sometimes fail to produce spermatozoa. The doctor may also ask whether any abdominal operations have been performed, such as a hernia repair; this is because, just as in women, the formation of adhesions (bands of scar tissue) or the development of infections following an operation can impair fertility. He or she will also inquire whether the man has had diseases such as mumps, or venereal diseases such as gonorrhoea and syphilis; these infections sometimes produce sterility by destroying the sperm-producing tissue of the testes or blocking the ducts which convey the sperm out of the testes.

Environmental factors may be relevant: for example, living for long periods at high altitudes has been shown to interfere with the production of spermatozoa. The doctor will also ask whether the man has been exposed to radiation or drugs, and whether his occupation involves contact with chemicals or exposure to high temperatures. General physical condition is also important, and sperm production may be unsatisfactory if the man is an invalid, grossly obese or a heavy drinker and/or smoker. Wearing tight-fitting underpants is thought to raise the normal scrotal temperature, which has a deleterious effect on the sperm.

If no abnormality to account for a low sperm count is discovered, blood tests may be performed to rule out a hormonal cause of the problem, although these often prove to be normal. If so, the man may simply be recommended to wear loose-fitting underpants and to apply occasional cold douches to the scrotum. These simple measures are sometimes sufficient to improve the sperm count. The doctor will also inquire whether the man believes he has made a woman pregnant in the past, and if any significant events have taken place since that time to account for the apparent loss of fertility (for example, a mumps infection).

The physical examination

The second step will be a physical examination. In the majority of men this reveals no cause of infertility, but an explanation will be found in a few cases. Poor body-hair growth or underdeveloped genitals may indicate a hormone deficiency; this can be confirmed by a measurement of hormone levels in the blood and in some cases hormone treatment may be recommended (see later in this chapter). The physical examination may also reveal that the testes have not descended into the scrotum and may be found in the groin, or indeed may be found to be completely absent and are presumed to be within the abdomen. Where this is discovered, an operation to remove the testes is recommended; the chances that they would ever produce spermatozoa are extremely limited, and if they are left in the abdomen there is a risk of malignant tumours developing in them.

On rare occasions, maldevelopment of the penis and/or scrotum may be a possible cause of infertility. An example is hypospadias, a condition in which the tube conducting the urine and sperm along the penis (the urethra) opens along the shaft of the penis and not at its end. There is a chance, therefore, that the ejaculate will not be deposited sufficiently high in the vagina.

Possibly a far more common cause of male infertility is a varicocele. It is an abnormality of the blood vessels within the scrotum around the testis. They become widely dilated and tortuous and appear as an enlarged area of the scrotum which, on palpation, feels like 'a bag of worms'. The man will be examined standing up when the doctor searches for a possible varicocele.

A varicocele is most commonly seen on the left side of the scrotum; the significance of this is possibly related to the arrangement of the venous system within the abdomen, although nobody is absolutely sure. Whatever the reason, the abnormally high blood flow through the scrotum (which can be measured scientifically using the technique of thermography) has the effect of raising the temperature around the testes, and although sperm motility, quality and density may be normal, it is thought that the raised temperature has an important effect on the sperm enzyme systems (the substances which control biochemical reactions within the spermatozoa themselves). I should point out that, as with everything to do with male infertility, varicoceles do not behave in a completely predictable fashion, and approximately two-thirds of men who have one are not infertile. However, in those who are thought to be infertile the treatment of a

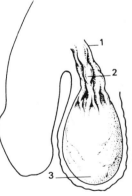

1 *Vas deferens*
2 *Varicocele*
3 *Testis*

varicocele should be given high priority. A minor operation is performed to tie off or remove the varicocele. The results of the operation are variable, with subsequent pregnancy rates of up to 55 per cent being claimed.

The general examination of the man may reveal some other disease which could affect fertility such as diabetes (which can cause impotence) or tuberculosis (which can occur in the scrotum, damaging the sperm-producing tissue, as well as in the lungs, spine, and kidneys), although these are serious diseases which would normally be detected long before a man is investigated for infertility.

The course of further investigations

The results of the seminalysis, medical history, and the physical examination will determine the course of further investigations of the man and subsequent treatment, if any. If no definite cause of infertility is discovered, the man may be offered more complex tests, but this depends very much on the facilities available to the investigating doctor. Whereas in the investigation of female infertility clear trends in tests and treatment emerge, and a woman would be examined and treated in a similar manner by different doctors, there are much greater gaps in our understanding of male infertility, and methods of treatment are in many cases still experimental. Thus it is difficult to predict the course of further investigation of the man would take. But if it is not possible for me to describe a step-by-step sequence of tests, I can illustrate some of the problems that crop up in male infertility and describe the various methods of treatment available.

Very roughly, and for the sake of convenience, we can divide the men who are still under investigation into two camps: those whose sperm count is low, and those whose is not. It is an artificial and by no means clearcut distinction, of course, and in practice it may have no bearing on the sequence of tests. (I have already pointed out that the sperm count is not always a reliable indicator of fertility.) But for convenience we can use this distinction to complete our review of male infertility. Firstly, I should like to consider those areas of infertility where the sperm count is *not* the critical factor, and then go on to those where the investigations are broadly concerned with discovering the cause of a low sperm count and attempting to improve it.

Where the sperm count seems satisfactory, the critical factor will be how the spermatozoa fare inside the woman's body: how they progress from the vagina through the cervix to the uterus and Fallopian tubes.

A number of tests can be performed to assess how the man's spermatozoa function once they are inside his partner's body, notably the postcoital test, which we have already mentioned. But before looking at this I will outline once again how fertilization occurs, as this will help to put the postcoital test into context.

Fertilization and the role of the cervical mucus

Placing the tip of the penis high in the vagina during intercourse ensures that the ejaculate is deposited at the neck of the womb (cervix). The spermatozoa then penetrate a plug of mucus which fills the small opening of the cervical canal into the cavity of the uterus (womb). This a very important process: complex chemical changes, known as capacitation, are believed to occur as the spermatozoa travel through the plug of mucus and the rest of the female reproductive tract, which greatly affect their chances of combining successfully with an ovum.

The plug of mucus forms a protective barrier to stop bacteria and other germs from entering the uterus. From the inner opening (os) of the cervix the spermatozoa quickly find themselves at the top (fundus) of the uterus. It is unlikely that they swim this distance; it is far more likely that they are squeezed up to the top by frequent contractions of the uterus. Once at the fundus, the spermatozoa pass along the Fallopian tubes. If they encounter an ovum (which will be much larger than them), the spermatozoa cluster around it, pressing their heads against its surface. Eventually one spermatozoon, and only one, penetrates the ovum.

The postcoital test

I have already described this procedure in Chapter 3. However, it is logical to mention it again in the context of male infertility, since although it is the woman who visits the doctor for the test, it is just as much a test of the man's fertility as it is of hers. In fact it provides a useful assessment of the couple's *combined* fertility by enabling the doctor to examine how well the man's spermatozoa survive in the woman's body. This is a very important point—in a number of infertile couples both partners are found to be perfectly normal and apparently fertile, but for various reasons the spermatozoa do not survive, or lose their motility and become sluggish, when they come into contact with the cervical mucus. This is often referred to as 'combined factor infertility'.

In the postcoital test, a small sample of cervical mucus is taken for examination within a few hours of intercourse. Under the microscope the doctor can see whether spermatozoa are present, how many there are, and whether they are active (motile) or dead. In most cases, seminalysis will already have been performed and the doctor will know the man's sperm count, and therefore the question of whether the spermatozoa are active or dead becomes far more important than their numbers. In general, if the results of the postcoital test are repeatedly good, that is, if the spermatozoa are seen to be moving freely in the cervical mucus, further investigations will concentrate on possible causes of infertility in the woman. But if the majority of spermatozoa are not moving about freely in the mucus, the chances of a pregnancy are low, and the reasons for the poor result must be investigated.

There are several reasons why the cervical mucus might be hostile to the spermatozoa. First, the mucus might be too acid, or there might not be enough of it. Spermatozoa are happiest in a slightly alkaline environment. The quantity of mucus secreted by the cervix, and its pH (degree of acidity or alkalinity) varies throughout the menstrual cycle. It is most alkaline and most abundant at the time of ovulation—i.e., at the most favourable time for conception, just when it is essential for the spermatozoa to survive in it and pass through it into the uterus. So one reason that the result of the postcoital test might be poor is that it was performed at the wrong time of the cycle—it should be done around the time of ovulation. If, however, the test is performed at the correct time and the mucus is still found to be too scanty, its quality and alkalinity may be improved by giving the woman oestrogen hormones during the first half of the menstrual cycle, although the effectiveness of this measure is often disappointing.

The second reason for a poor postcoital test result is infections of the cervix, in which case the mucus might be cloudy in appearance. Appropriate antibiotics will be prescribed, and the postcoital test repeated after the infection has cleared up.

A third reason is that the spermatozoa themselves may be abnormal or defective in some way. However, this would normally have been noticed during seminalysis, and further investigations prescribed as necessary at that stage.

The fourth and most significant reason for poor sperm motility in the cervical mucus is the presence of antibodies.

Sperm antibodies

It has been known since the beginning of the twentieth century that the body can produce antibodies against human spermatozoa. Antibodies are substances that circulate in the blood and body tissues and which help the body to destroy foreign 'invaders'. They are manufactured by certain types of white blood cell and form an important part of the immune system—our defence mechanism against infection. Normally the antigens (invading substances which spark off the production of antibodies) are disease-causing organisms such as bacteria or viruses. But certain women produce antibodies against their partner's spermatozoa. We do not yet understand how this happens. In fact it might be more accurate to say that we do not yet understand how it is that in the normal course of events a woman's body does *not* respond to spermatozoa as it would to other 'foreign' cells, that is, by producing antibodies! But whatever the mechanism involved, if a woman produces antibodies against the man's sperm, fertility is likely to be impaired. At the postcoital test adequate numbers of sperm will be seen, but they will be dead, having been immobilized by the antibodies, and therefore incapable of fertilizing an ovum.

It is perhaps more surprising to discover that the seminal fluid of some men contains antibodies against their own spermatozoa. In fact, spermatozoa are antigenically different from the man who produces them (i.e., they are likely to stimulate an antibody reaction), but normally special cells protect them from being exposed to the immune system. If there is some breakdown in this mechanism, antibodies may appear in the man's blood and sometimes in the genital secretions. These antibodies can render the spermatozoa ineffective by causing them to agglutinate (clump together). Other agglutinins (agglutinating substances) are found in the seminal fluid of a few infertile men, but are never seen in fertile men.

Various tests can be performed to follow up the postcoital test to confirm evidence of the presence of antibodies. The most important of these is the sperm–cervical mucus contact test, or SCMC. This consists of mixing a tiny drop of the man's semen with a little of the cervical mucus taken from the woman just before the time of ovulation, and examining the mixture under a microscope. When antibodies are present the spermatozoa are seen to display a shaking or jerking movement, quite distinct from the normal progressive movement through the mucus. Repeating the test using semen from a donor can identify which partner may be producing antibodies.

Treatments

There are several possible modes of treatment for anti-sperm antibodies, none of which is entirely satisfactory. Antibodies are sometimes produced by men with an infection of the prostate gland; long–term administration of antibiotics can result in a significant decrease in the number of antibodies, and some pregnancies have been achieved following this treatment. A few successes have also been achieved by 'washing' the spermatozoa free of the antibodies in the laboratory and then introducing them into the woman's uterus by artificial insemination or by in vitro fertilization. Treatment with anti–flammatory hormones (steroids) may also succeed in reducing the number of antibodies and produce occasional pregnancies.

There we shall leave our discussion of antibodies and other factors affecting the survival of spermatozoa inside the woman's body. This is one of the areas of infertility into which the most intensive research is being done, and we must hope that as knowledge of the subject increases, so the outlook for infertile couples with these particular problems will brighten. Now we shall move on to tests and treatment aimed at improving the fertility of men with a low sperm count.

Biopsy of the testicles

Some surgeons offer the infertile man, in whom no obvious cause of infertility has been found, a testicular biopsy and exploration. The object of this is to rule out the possibility of disease or obstruction inside the testes. In a small operation, the scrotum is opened and the testes are examined for evidence of serious infection, such as mumps or syphilis. A small snippet of tissue may be taken from the testis (a biopsy) and sent to the pathological laboratory for analysis. A careful search will also be made for blocked tubes within the testis: a common site for such obstruction is the epididymis. The testicular biopsy may well yield information about the state of sperm production within the testis, although, disappointingly, testicular biopsies are often normal and give no clue to the cause of infertility. In addition, the abnormalities which are found often cannot be corrected, and there is a small but definite risk that sperm production may be suppressed after a testicular biopsy.

Where an obstruction is found, particularly of the epididymis, an effort to open up the blockage is made in an operation known as a vasoepididymostomy. However, the extremely poor results of this operation suggest that there is a deficiency in sperm transport which may be related to abnormalities of the lining of the tube rather than the blocked passage alone—as in the case of the Fallopian tubes (see p. 118).

Drug treatment

In recent years there has been remarkable interest in drug treatment for male infertility. However, little real progress has so far been made, although the amount of research conducted throughout the world does give considerable hope for the near future. Improvement in fertility is sometimes achieved by giving extra male sex hormones (androgens). Their effects, however, are sometimes paradoxical and one such androgen, known as mesterolone, produces improved sperm counts in half the patients to whom it is given, while the other half show decreased counts.

Another treatment involves the stimulation of the sperm-producing cells by the natural hormone from the pituitary known as follicle-stimulating hormone (FSH). Repeated injections of this hormone have proved to be of some benefit in patients who produce low numbers of spermatozoa. Further research is currently being conducted into the use of clomiphene in male infertility following its success in female infertility. At present, however, the extent of its usefulness in the male is not clear, and the same is true of another drug used in the treatment of female infertility, bromocriptine. In this respect attempts at therapy are hampered by our limited understanding of the normal process of sperm production, function and transport.

The role of hormones

Much of the current research into male infertility centres on the role of hormones, and it may be useful for us to look more closely at this subject; although it is fairly technical, most people find it intriguing. For those who are not certain about what the function of these much-talked-about substances is, hormones can be described as chemical messenger substances which are carried around the body in the bloodstream. They are released by the endocrine glands, which act in close conjunction with the nervous system; the major hormone-secreting glands are the pituitary, thyroid and parathyroid glands, pancreas, adrenals, ovaries and testes. The effect of hormones is long-term stimulation of other glands and organs in the body. For example, hormones released by the thyroid gland control the rate of metabolism, the process by which energy is made available. In this way hormones are involved in the control of all the vital internal processes of the body, including those that concern us here—the function of the reproductive organs.

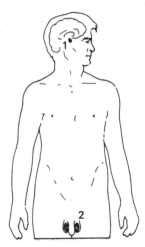

Endocrinal glands which produce hormones affecting male fertility. 1 Pituitary 2 Testes.

We have already seen that the pituitary gland in the brain produces follicle-stimulating hormone (FSH) which controls the amount of spermatozoa produced. FSH does not actually speed up sperm production, which has been shown to be a biologically constant process; what it is thought to do is to decrease the number of early sperm cells that degenerate during sperm production and thereby effect an increased output of spermatozoa. If the pituitary fails to produce FSH, testicular function will be poor. However, it has been estimated that in men who approach their doctors about infertility, FSH deficiency is a causative factor in less than 0.5 per cent of cases.

However, it is useful to measure the level of FSH circulating in the blood, because it provides a fair guide to the condition of the sperm-producing parts of the testes and bears a direct relationship to the sperm density of the patient. If the testes are producing insufficient spermatozoa, the pituitary gland will respond by secreting more and more FSH in an attempt to stimulate sperm production. Finding raised levels of FSH in the blood of men with either no or very little sperm production (less than 5 million per ml) indicates that the sperm-producing parts of the testes may well be severely damaged. Conversely, a very low sperm count with a normal concentration of FSH in the blood would indicate that the absence of sperm in the ejaculate is probably due to an obstruction of the duct system, which may possibly be cleared by surgery. In many clinics, therefore, the measurement of FSH has gradually replaced the use of testicular biopsy as an indicator of the state of sperm-producing parts of the testes in men with very low sperm counts. When FSH levels are found to be either abnormally raised or lowered, however, it is usual to make repeat measurements, as the pituitary secretes FSH in bursts rather than constantly.

Other hormone measurements

Other hormones which are sometimes measured in the investigation of male infertility are luteinizing hormone (LH), which, like FSH, is secreted by the pituitary, and testosterone, the principal male sex hormone, which is produced by the testes themselves. LH stimulates special cells in the testes, known as Leydig cells, to produce testosterone, which is necessary for sperm development. Variations in the levels of these hormones may give further information about the nature of the damage to the testes which could be causing the infertility.

Another pituitary hormone whose role in both male and female infertility is under investigation is called prolactin; its effects are not completely understood. It is known that a raised prolactin concentration in men is usually associated with impotence rather than sperm failure itself. Prolactin concentrations in men with low sperm counts have been described as normal by some researchers and as raised by others. More encouraging are the recent reports that some men with raised prolactin levels in their blood and very low sperm counts have had their sperm counts improved by the use of the drug bromocriptine, which has the effect of lowering the level of prolactin. However, the number of patients so far treated is small, and further information is necessary before accurate predictions can be made about the use of this drug in male infertility.

Hormone treatments

The number of patients with FSH deficiency is not very large, as I mentioned earlier. Nevertheless, treatment by giving injections of FSH has been successful in some cases. The treatment may have to be continued for many months and injections of FSH are extremely expensive. Hormone deficiencies are not found in many infertile men, but in spite of this there is a great temptation to stimulate the testis hormonally anyway. A number of studies have been performed, but unfortunately the information they have provided has on the whole been inadequate.

Stimulation of the testes is attempted either by giving injections of FSH or by giving the anti-oestrogen drug clomiphene. A certain number of patients do respond to treatment with these agents, but owing to the long duration of the sperm-production cycle (70 days) the treatment must be continued for periods of up to six months. It is not possible to predict whether or not a patient will respond to this sort of treatment, but most experts agree that little benefit is obtained by patients with either no sperm production or sperm production that is extremely limited.

Another hormone treatment, which has been tried out in a considerable number of patients, consists of injections of testosterone. This has the effect of suppressing sperm production, and the hope is that when treatment is stopped, sperm counts will rise ('rebound') to higher concentrations than before treatment was started. In a study performed in 1975, 131 men with reduced sperm counts were treated with 'rebound testosterone therapy' and a pregnancy rate of 29 per cent was reported during the rebound phase. However, this high rate of success has not been achieved by many other studies.

It is difficult to contemplate that major advances in the treatment of male infertility will be made until after many fundamental questions about the subject have been answered more fully. Improvement in sperm production by manipulation of the hormonal environment in fairly random fashion is probably meeting the limited success that almost any arbitrary form of treatment can achieve, and we do not properly understand the underlying problems which need correction.

For the man with adequate sperm production the field of immunology, and antibody interactions in particular, would seem to be yielding the sort of answers which might assist therapy. For the man with nil or extremely limited sperm production, the outlook remains bleak.

I wonder if the pressures on the medical profession and organizations are sufficiently strong to ensure that adequate effort and interest are being applied to the subject of male infertility. I suspect not. It is easy to appreciate that the recent innovations and improvements in the management of female infertility have encouraged deep interest in the subject among professionals and public alike. No such strides have been made in male infertility recently and the field may well be under-researched at present, which hardly stimulates vast numbers of doctors to take up interest in the subject.

Perhaps the time is not ripe. Male infertility has yet to become the subject of cocktail party gossip in the same way as sex (both hetero- and homosexual), politics, illness, religion and death. One assumes that the almost indissoluble association between male infertility and impotence prevents the strong lobby in social, medical and governmental circles needed to bring the extent of the problem to light and encourage more research and treatment centres.

In the meantime many men will be walking away from infertility investigations after having been told that there is little or nothing, given the present state of knowledge, that can be done for them. To a man brought up with the common supposition that infertility always occurs because the woman is 'barren', this comes as a great shock. He will know that his sexual prowess is not at fault—he will have been assured that the problem is common among all sorts of men—and he will know that probably nothing he has

The future for male infertility

done in the past has caused his infertility. One thing for sure is that he will need tremendous help from his partner as he accepts this catastrophe in his life. Perhaps this may possibly be a time to consider artificial insemination by donor (see p.144). This is most definitely not the time for blame or recrimination, but the time 'for better, for worse'—for love and support.

5

More complicated tests

When the woman returns for her second interview with the doctor, the results of the temperature charts, postcoital test and seminalysis are usually at hand, and some planning of further investigations, if required, can be made accordingly.

First, if the temperature charts show that intercourse is not taking place at the optimum time, further advice can be given by the doctor and a further period of 'trying', say four months, will be recommended without any further tests during that time.

Second, if the sperm count is very low and there is doubt about the man's fertility, he might be referred for specialized tests and treatment (described in the previous chapter). However, if the sperm count is low but there is also some evidence that the woman is not ovulating properly (from the temperature charts, for instance) it will be worthwhile treating her first and attempting to get her ovulating regularly before sending the man for investigations. There are two reasons for this: firstly, even with a low sperm count a man can be quite fertile, and if treatment can succeed in inducing the woman to ovulate, she might just conceive; secondly, as you can see from the previous chapter, there is disappointingly little that can be done for the majority of infertile men, so the best hope for conception is to get the woman ovulating properly and hope that the man's sperm will be sufficient to fertilize her ova. What I am trying to say is that if you have a couple where both the man and the woman have 'marginal' fertility, it is in general easier at the moment to improve the woman's fertility than it is to improve the man's.

If, however, seminalysis shows that the man is not producing any spermatozoa at all and a blood test shows high levels of follicle-stimulating hormone (FSH), it is not worthwhile proceeding with more complex tests on the woman. The high hormone levels usually indicate that the sperm-producing tissues of the testes are damaged; the pituitary gland is sending out unusually large amounts of FSH in an attempt to stimulate the inactive testes. If this is the case, there is little hope of restoring the man's fertility. One solution the couple might wish to contemplate is artificial insemination by donor (see p. 144), and if so the doctor may wish to perform further tests to establish that the woman is ovulating regularly.

Failure of ovulation

Let us now deal with the 20–25 per cent of women who are infertile as a result of problems with ovulation. Evidence that ovulation is not regular, or even completely absent, might come from a history of scanty, irregular or absent menstrual periods, or from temperature charts and the other tests (examination of cervical mucus, endometrial biopsy, etc.) already mentioned. To eliminate any doubt as to whether ovulation is occurring a 'serum progesterone' measurement must be taken. This is simply an analysis of the level of the hormone progesterone in the bloodstream. After ovulation has occurred the level of progesterone rises in order to prepare the womb lining (endometrium) and the rest of the body for the pregnancy which may follow. The endometrium becomes secretory and ready to receive a fertilized egg. The increased progesterone levels can be measured by a simple blood test, usually performed on the 21st day of the cycle. If the ovum is not fertilized the level of hormone falls again, the menstrual period begins, and the endometrium and about 50 to 150 ml of blood are shed. So if the serum progesterone is satisfactorily raised it can be assumed that ovulation really has taken place, and if it is not, the doctor can be worried that ovulation has not occurred.

If it is found that the periods are irregular or scanty, more regular ovulation can usually be induced by giving one of the 'fertility drugs', which I discuss in chapter 8. However, where the woman is not menstruating at all matters are a little more complex, and a series of tests to rule out serious causes is usually performed.

Those women who have never had regular, satisfactory periods, or who have never menstruated, usually consult their doctors before marrying and seeking advice for infertility. Most of the women undergoing investigations for infertility are between 20 and 40 years of age and if a woman does not begin to menstruate properly she is usually investigated by her doctor before she reaches the age of 20, although one or two will slip through. These women include the few with chromosomal defects and rare congenital abnormalities, such as failure of the ovaries or uterus to develop properly. I will not deal with these cases further as the problems and their investigations are often complex and are beyond the scope of this book.

The majority of women with ovulation problems who seek help for infertility will probably have menstruated normally, or almost normally, at some time in their lives; the periods may then have stopped (say after discontinuing the contraceptive pill) or become irregular or scanty.

As mentioned before, where there are ovulation problems of any kind it is usual to perform some screening tests such as a chest x-ray, skull x-ray (with special views to examine the little 'cellar' at the base of the skull where the pituitary gland lies), tests of adrenal, pituitary, and thyroid function, as well as blood-sugar tests to exclude diabetes.

The effect of excess prolactin

In recent years a very important screening test has been introduced. It has been found that a few women produce an excess of a hormone from the pituitary gland called prolactin. (Prolactin is the hormone, released after childbirth, which stimulates the glands in the breast to produce milk.) In some women this abnormally high prolactin level in the blood causes the breasts to secrete a little fluid and interfere with the periods. Other women have raised prolactin levels without breast discharge and period problems. The prolactin level can be measured by a blood test. An excess of prolactin is frequently associated with a small tumour of the pituitary gland, and so skull x-rays and scans are ordered immediately if a raised prolactin level is found. And now for the good news: a drug called bromocriptine is now available which can lower raised prolactin levels, so that infertility resulting from such raised levels can be reversed. Many pregnancies have been made possible by this drug in the last decade.

During pregnancy and, of course, breast feeding, prolactin levels rise considerably. If the pituitary gland has a small prolactin-secreting tumour inside it and a pregnancy is achieved, then this tumour will probably enlarge further and even press on the optic nerves, causing partial or even total blindness. It is therefore very important to investigate and deal with any suspected pituitary tumour properly before the woman with high levels of prolactin in her blood is allowed to become pregnant.

I hope I have not lost you with this digression. I was saying that supplementary tests are usually performed when ovulation problems are suspected, and if failure of ovulation is confirmed then specific treatment to induce ovulation is commenced. Of course, if the supplementary tests reveal some more general disorder, for example, thyroid disease, this will be treated and the periods then observed for the return of normal ovulation.

As mentioned in the last chapter, arrangements are usually made to perform the postcoital test early on. Adequate spermatozoal function, as revealed by the postcoital test, should be established before the next series of investigations on the woman, which become a little more involved.

If ovulation is satisfactory

Let us assume that the 'non-ovulators' have been sorted out and their problems are being treated (see later); this still leaves a large proportion of women who will need further tests to identify the cause of their problem. But don't forget that quite a few women will go through the complete series of investigations and no cause of infertility will be found, and that, as stated earlier, many of these will subsequently become pregnant without help.

Endometriosis

Endometriosis is a fairly common condition which in certain women might be high on the doctor's list of suspicions, if ovulation is satisfactory, but they fail to conceive. Very simply, specks or blobs of endometrial cells (the cells lining the inside of the uterus) can appear elsewhere—inside the muscle of the uterus, on the ovaries,

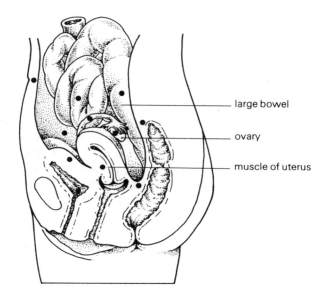

— large bowel

— ovary

— muscle of uterus

Typical sites of endometriosis: abnormal patches of endometrial cells which apparently migrate from the lining of the uterus to other parts of the abdomen.

and even on the surface of other pelvic organs such as the bladder and large bowel. Like the cells inside the womb, these abnormal blobs of endometrium respond to the hormones produced during the menstrual cycle—they enlarge and may even bleed a little at period times. The periods are affected—they may be prolonged and irregular, and painful too. Endometriosis tends to occur in women who are in their 30s and early 40s, and occasionally those under 30 years of age. These women usually have not had a pregnancy. The effects on fertility of even a few endometriotic spots in the pelvis can be marked (and until relatively recently these effects had been underestimated or overlooked; doctors are very aware of this problem nowadays).

So a woman in her 20s or 30s who has irregular, painful periods, and on examination has tenderness and thickening of the supporting ligaments of the uterus, might well be suspected of having endometriosis. The diagnosis is usually confirmed at laparoscopy (see p. 89) when these spots can be seen. Of course the woman may also have some other cause for her infertility, such as blocked tubes, and this will be checked too, but most doctors on discovering endometriosis during infertility investigations will want to treat it, as many women will become pregnant after treatment if this condition is the sole cause of their problem. As many women, especially working women, are tending to delay starting their families until their late 20s and 30s, endometriosis as a cause of infertility might become more and more common.

Why do these 'blobs' appear in the pelvis? Well, that is a good question to which there are several possible answers, and these may be only partly true. Probably the most easily understood and popular explanation is the 'retrograde menstruation' theory—that cells from the lining of the womb pass upwards into the Fallopian tubes and out into the pelvic cavity, where they settle down, perhaps on the bowel or bladder. These cells produce powerful hormone-like substances called prostaglandins, and these may interfere with the ovum after ovulation. This simple explanation will have to suffice. There are many questions about endometriosis still to be answered but an important fact is now at hand. Elaborate studies in both the United States and the United Kingdom have shown that even a small area of endometriosis, just a few black speckles (which are described as resembling a 'powder burn' from a gun), can exert a profound effect on fertility in some women, and therefore needs treatment. The treatment of this condition will be dealt with later (see p. 113), but two last points are worthy of mention. Firstly, remember that all women with endometriosis are not necessarily infertile; secondly, not all women who have irregular, painful periods in their 30s and 40s will necessarily have endometriosis—although some will, and will benefit from treatment.

The Fallopian tubes

This is the next big question to be resolved after a woman is shown to be ovulating: are the Fallopian tubes blocked, and if they are not, are the lining cells working properly, or are they damaged? As has been discussed before, at ovulation the ovum is released on to the surface of the ovary and enters the Fallopian tube, which conducts the ovum along its length, so that it can enter the uterus. If the ovum is fertilized, it stays in the tube for two or three days before passing down into the uterus for implantation. It is easy to see that the tube is more than just a pipeline carrying the ovum from ovary to uterus; the delicate ovum is nurtured, protected and guided for several days by the cells lining the Fallopian tube.

The tubes are a very important factor in infertility. The delicate lining of the tube, and indeed the whole tube itself, can be seriously damaged by infection, especially if the infection goes untreated or is treated inadequately at the time. Scarring can result from these infections, although not, of course, in every case. High on the list of infections which can cause tube damage is the venereal disease gonorrhoea. Much more uncommonly, tuberculosis can infect the Fallopian tubes. Infection following surgery to the bowel, e.g., appendicectomy, may also affect the tube and perhaps bind it down in adhesions (bands of scar tissue). An ectopic pregnancy in the tube may have been removed in the past, along with a portion of tube. And a woman may have been sterilized and her tubes cut, cauterized or clipped by a surgeon—this topic is covered in Chapter 10. A history of pelvic infection will also focus the doctor's attention on the state of the Fallopian tubes.

The first line of investigation will be to see if the tubes are opened or blocked. A rather old-fashioned test is still occasionally used for this; it is called insufflation.

Insufflation

In this procedure, also known as Rubin's test, a small hollow tube (*cannula*) is inserted into the uterus through the vagina, an air-tight seal being achieved around the cervix. Gas, usually carbon dioxide, is passed into the uterus, up along both Fallopian tubes, and out into the abdominal cavity. The pressure of the gas is recorded. In addition a stethoscope is placed low down on the woman's abdomen on both left and right so that the gas can be heard bubbling out of the tubes. Carbon dioxide is usually used as this is absorbed quickly into the bloodstream and then exhaled through the lungs, as in normal respiration. Pain may be felt in the shoulder as a result of gas collecting in the abdomen and irritating the nerves supplying the diaphragm; the shoulder is supplied by the same nerves. This 'referred pain' can help to establish whether a Fallopian tube is open.

If no gas can be heard issuing from the tubes and the

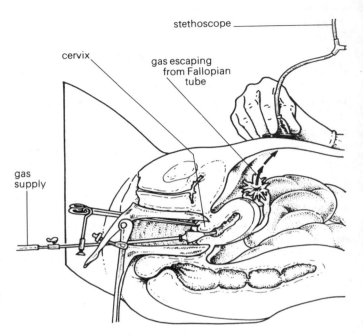

stethoscope

cervix

gas escaping
from Fallopian
tube

gas
supply

*The technique of insufflation.
If the Fallopian tubes are
patent (open), gas is heard
escaping from them through a
stethoscope held to the
abdomen.*

pressure remains fairly high then it is assumed that both tubes are blocked. If gas cannot be heard over one side and the pressure is moderately elevated, it is assumed that one of the tubes is blocked. Occasionally, the pressure may wax and wane and this might be due to spasm of the tubes. It was a popular idea some years ago that such tubal spasm might account for the anxiety and tension element in the subfertility of some women. It was thought that the point could be demonstrated by giving suitable muscle relaxants during insufflation. While this is an appealing idea, and may contain some truth, its popularity has declined somewhat recently.

Advantages of insufflation lie in its simplicity and safety, while the main disadvantage is the paucity and quality of the information it provides. When describing it above I used the term 'assumed' as indeed all evidence is inferior to the eye-witness account. Insufflation may tell the doctor that there is a blockage in one or both tubes, but it does not locate whereabouts in the tube the blockage is, and more importantly, it does not give any indication about the state of the tubes or the extent of the damage, which is important if tubal surgery is to be considered. Insufflation has been largely superseded by laparoscopy.

If the doctor suspects that there might be some develop- **Hysterosalpingogram** mental or other abnormality of the uterus and/or the Fallopian tubes he or she might suggest an x-ray investigation called a 'hysterosalpingogram' (based on the Greek words for womb, tube and picture). Most doctors refer to it as an HSG for short. What sort of abnormalities do we have in mind? Clues might be obtained from the medical history and pelvic examination. It is extremely rare for a woman to be born without a uterus, but occasionally women are discovered to have only one Fallopian tube. Rarely, the uterus has not developed sufficiently in size (hypoplastic uterus) and is not capable of holding a pregnancy within. Any woman with one congenital abnormality in her body may have more and these may involve the reproductive organs. A woman who has had repeated miscarriages may have an abnormally shaped womb which needs investigating. A womb severely distorted by fibroids might also be revealed by an HSG.

An HSG is usually performed with the patient awake, although a few doctors do it with the patient under a general anaesthetic. The procedure is not without some discomfort, but usually does not produce severe pain. Once again a hollow tube is inserted into the cervical canal and a fluid-tight seal against the cervix is obtained. A radiopaque liquid (which shows up on an x-ray film) is gently injected into the uterus, while the pelvis is observed under an x-ray image intensifier, which looks like a TV screen. The liquid fills the uterus and outlines its inner shape. This filling can cause cramping, like an intense menstrual cramp.

The liquid is then observed as it goes into the tubes, along their length and spills into the abdominal cavity. The site of any blockage can be noted and abnormalities in the shape of the womb and tubes discovered too. One or two still-picture x-rays are taken for the record. The actual filming takes two or three minutes, but the time taken for the whole procedure is about 10 minutes and is occasionally combined with an endometrial biopsy. Every precaution, however, must be taken beforehand to ensure that the woman is not pregnant at the time of the HSG.

What an HSG can detect

The uterus is formed in the first two months of fetal life by the fusion of two tubes. If that fusion is totally incomplete a double uterus will be formed. If the fusion is partial a rudimentary horn or bicornuate (two-horned) uterus may result. These abnormalities, which can be discoverd by HSG, do not cause infertility in every case by any means, but in a very few women they do, and may need corrective surgery, which is discussed in Chapter 9.

The site of any blockage of the tubes (or at least the blockage nearest to the uterus) will be shown up by the HSG, but as with insufflation, there is little information given about the state of the tubes themselves. If the blockage is very close to the uterus the rest of the tube will not be shown up at all by the HSG. If infection and/or adhesions have damaged the tube, but not completely blocked it, it will have a 'kinked' appearance, but this only shows up very occasionally. It is because of this limitation of information that the HSG has been largely replaced by laparoscopy. However, it is still useful in cases where uterine abnormalities are suspected and for locating the site of tubal blockages close to where the tubes join the uterus (cornua).

Finally, as with many procedures in infertility work, it sometimes happens that an HSG is followed by a pregnancy. Many radiologists and gynaecologists can quote dozens of examples where a woman has conceived soon after having an HSG. (A radiologist is a doctor who specializes in the study and analysis of x-ray pictures, not to be confused with the radiographer, who is the person who takes the pictures and processes them for the radiologist.) This subsequent pregnancy may be due to the relief of anxiety a normal HSG result can produce, or it may be that the oily radiopaque liquid used may 'flush away the cobwebs' in the tubes. It may be true that tiny adhesions inside the tubes that in some cases are responsible for infertility may be divided by the HSG liquid. While this is a very welcome side effect for the lucky few women who enjoy a pregnancy assisted in some way by an HSG, it must be emphasized that the HSG is primarily an

The hysterosalpingogram

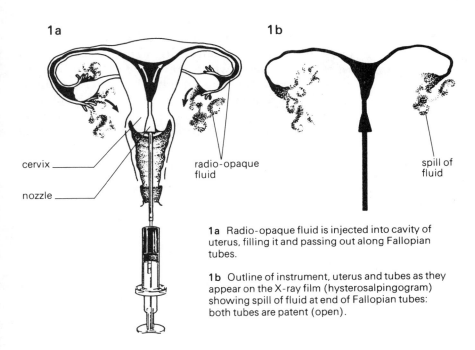

cervix

nozzle

radio-opaque fluid

spill of fluid

1a Radio-opaque fluid is injected into cavity of uterus, filling it and passing out along Fallopian tubes.

1b Outline of instrument, uterus and tubes as they appear on the X-ray film (hysterosalpingogram) showing spill of fluid at end of Fallopian tubes: both tubes are patent (open).

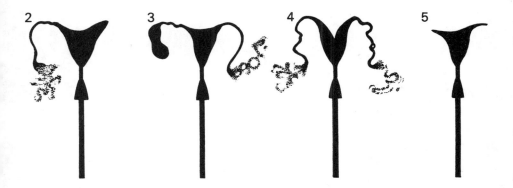

2 Right-hand Fallopian tube is open but left tube blocked at entrance to uterus.

3 Right-hand tube is sac-like and blocked (hydrosalpinx).

4 Both tubes are open but uterus has a divided cavity (septate or bicornuate uterus).

5 Right tube is blocked close to uterus, left tube blocked half way along its length.

investigation and not a treatment!

Those women who are found to have blocked tubes after insufflation or an HSG may be helped by surgery. Before offering any such operation a gynaecologist will want to see the state of the tubes and the pelvis in general in order to assess the chances of success, or even to see whether it is worthwhile attempting surgery. For this reason, in women where tubal blockage is either suspected, or suggested by the other investigations mentioned, the majority of gynaecologists now choose laparoscopy, and this important investigation is covered in considerable detail in the next chapter.

6

Laparoscopy

In the last chapter we saw that if investigations show that **The laparoscope** the woman is ovulating and that the man has a satisfactory seminalysis, the next thing the investigating doctor will want to know is whether the woman's Fallopian tubes are blocked, and, in addition, what general condition they are in. He or she will also want to check for possible abnormalities of the uterus and ovaries. I have described two methods of testing for tubal blockage—insufflation and the hysterosalpingogram (HSG). The hysterosalpingogram is also useful for demonstrating uterine abnormalities. The main disadvantage of both these methods is that they are essentially indirect methods of inspection, and are obviously inferior to a direct method—where the doctor can actually see all the pelvic organs.

Direct inspection can be achieved by the use of an instrument called a laparoscope, the word means roughly 'a telescope in the abdomen', from the Greek *lapar*, loin or flank. Before the advent of the laparoscope, direct examination was only possible by cutting into, and formally opening up, the abdomen (laparotomy). This caused the patient not inconsiderable discomfort and a week or two in hospital afterwards. What was needed was some way of viewing the pelvic organs without having to make a large incision.

The idea of putting a telescope through the abdominal wall of an anaesthetized patient to examine his or her internal organs occurred to surgeons at around the turn of the century, but the idea had to wait for several major improvements in medicine before it could be put into practice. First, anaesthetics had to become smoother and safer. Second, some method of inflating the abdomen was needed to create a space around the organs so that the telescope could focus on them. These two main problems were overcome soon after World War II with improvements in anaesthesia, the use of muscle relaxants, and the introduction of the use of carbon dioxide or nitrous oxide (the 'laughing gas' used in simple anaesthetics) to inflate the abdomen. These particular gases are used because any remaining after the operation will be quickly and harmlessly absorbed into the bloodstream. The final breakthrough came with the introduction of fibre-optics. A fibre-optic rod, made of a special kind of glass fibre, can be used to transmit light down the telescope—thus providing good illumination of the area under examination without needing to use extra instruments involving bulbs and electric cables.

By the early 1960s the instrument was in use throughout the world and had proved highly rewarding in infertility work. (Its usefulness is by no means confined to infertility work, nor even to gynaecology; the laparoscope is often used to examine other abdominal organs.)

How laparoscopy is carried out

Laparoscopy is always performed in hospital; it can be carried out under a local anaesthetic but the procedure is usually quicker and offers little discomfort if performed under general anaesthesia, i.e., with the patient fully unconscious. A light premedication is given approximately one hour before the operation to make the patient feel relaxed and to dry the secretions in the mouth. Immediately before the operation the patient is given an injection into a vein on the back of the hand or arm which induces her to fall asleep within a few seconds. A second injection will be given to relax all the muscles of the body, and anaesthetic gases which keep the patient unconscious throughout the operation are passed into the lungs by means of either a soft tube passed between the vocal cords and down into the windpipe (trachea) or a close-fitting face mask. The patient's breathing movements are under the control of the anaesthetist, who stands at the head of the operating table and carefully monitors the breathing rate and volume, flow, and mixture of gases.

The patient is placed on the operating table and her legs

light beam   laparoscope

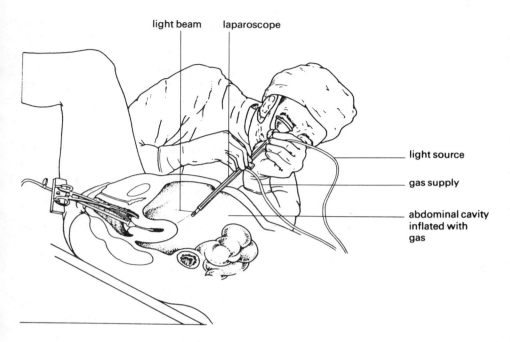

light source

gas supply

abdominal cavity
inflated with
gas

are raised in a pair of stirrups. The surface of the abdomen is cleansed, draped in sterile towels and a small tube (catheter) is inserted into the bladder through the urethra. All the urine is expelled by pressing the abdomen above the bladder. This is to make sure that the bladder is not distended, obscuring the view inside, and to avoid possible damage to it during the operation. The catheter is removed and a small incision is made into the skin just below the umbilicus (navel). A thin hollow needle (known as a Verres needle) is inserted through the incision into the peritoneal cavity (the space inside the inner lining layer of the abdominal wall). The needle is connected to a controlled supply of carbon dioxide or nitrous oxide gas which is passed into the abdomen slowly at around one to three litres per minute. This inflates the abdomen, raising the abdominal muscles away from the intestines and pelvic organs to produce a space in which the laparoscope can be manoeuvred with safety and ease.

When sufficient gas has been passed, usually three to four litres, the previously flat abdominal wall has become dome-shaped. The Verres needle is then removed. Since

Above: *During laparoscopy the surgeon can observe the Fallopian tubes as dye is squirted through the uterus and escapes through the Fallopian tubes.*

the muscles it passes through are fairly elastic and the hole it makes relatively small, the hole seals immediately and no gas is lost. Now the laparoscope is inserted. The instrument itself is simply a telescope—similar to ones used to inspect other areas of the body, such as the cystoscope, which is for examing the bladder, through the urethra. It is usually 5–10mm in diameter, and has a passage to keep a small flow of gas passing into the abdomen, replacing any losses, and a fibre-optic light source as mentioned before. The laparoscope is inserted through the incision in the abdomen and passed between the two vertical abdominal muscles which run from the pubic bone up to the chest. The patient has been tipped head down by tilting the operating table; this causes the intestines to slide downwards into the upper abdomen, leaving the pelvic organs relatively uncovered and easily visible.

While the patient is under the anaesthetic for laparoscopy, doctors usually take the opportunity to look for evidence to confirm or negate previous suggestions, such as an enlarged uterus. At this point a thin hollow probe is placed in the uterine canal to enable the uterus to be moved and dye to be injected along the Fallopian tubes.

What the doctor looks for

After passing the laparoscope into the abdomen the doctor looks through the eyepiece and takes a general view of the pelvis. The initial appearance may suggest previous pelvic infections (or even current infections), particularly by the presence of adhesions, which are rubbery bands of scar tissue binding one structure to another. A common site for these is the right side of the pelvis, where they may occur as a result of appendicitis. The bowel is observed, especially for signs of infection such as colitis and Crohn's disease (a chronic inflammatory condition of the bowel), and then the patient's head is tipped even further down by rotating the table, so that gravity pulls the mobile intestines down and away from the pelvis.

A good view of the uterus is obtained by moving it back and forth by means of the hollow intrauterine tube previously inserted through the vagina. A satisfactory round or pear-like shape is expected, and the doctor will be anxious to rule out any congenital abnormalities of the

Problems diagnosed by laparoscopy

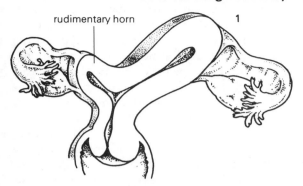

rudimentary horn

1 Unicornuate (one-horned) uterus. Incomplete fusion of the two primitive tubes in a developing fetus can produce this condition.

2 Fibroids (non-malignant tumours) can form in the uterine cavity, in the myometrium (muscle), or beneath the surface.

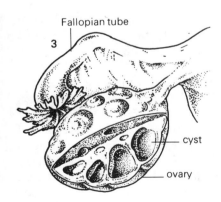

fibroids

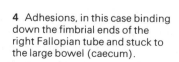

Fallopian tube

cyst

ovary

3 Polycystic ovaries. Multiple cysts form in the periphery of the ovary with excess stroma in between.

4 Adhesions, in this case binding down the fimbrial ends of the right Fallopian tube and stuck to the large bowel (caecum).

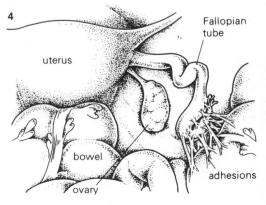

Fallopian tube

uterus

bowel

ovary

adhesions

types mentioned in the last chapter—such as bicornuate uterus (which results from incomplete development of the uterus in the fetus), unicornuate uterus with or without a rudimentary horn, or even a small, stunted (hypoplastic) uterus which would be totally incapable of sustaining a pregnancy. The uterine shape may commonly be distorted by the presence of fibroids—benign tumours of the uterine muscle. All the above conditions may be causes of infertility and will be carefully watched for.

The doctor will then turn to the state of the ovaries, indeed to see whether they are both present and have an appearance suggesting normal function. Absence of one ovary may be noted, but this is fairly rare, and in any case, provided that the other ovary is working normally, does not usually cause infertility. However, the doctor may see evidence of the 'polycystic ovary syndrome' (some of which will be of the Stein Leventhal type). In this condition, the ovaries are enlarged and polycystic (consisting of multiple cysts). The condition is associated with a failure to ovulate, but this can often be cured by surgery (wedge resection) or by one of the fertility drugs (see p. 105). Polycystic ovaries may appear relatively normal at laparoscopy—the diagnosis may then be made on the internal appearance of the ovaries by ultrasound scanning, along with hormone blood tests.

Ultrasound scanning is a means of imaging the ovaries on a video screen using harmless, painless sound waves. A full bladder is required during this examination to lift up the uterus and ovaries, and to provide accurate location of these organs as they lie against the bladder. The urine in the bladder appears as a large black area around which the organs lie, and can be identified. The ultrasound scan 'looks inside' the ovaries and shows how the follicles are arranged and allows the ultrasonographer to measure the follicles accurately. Polycystic ovaries may not appear abnormal when looked at by direct vision from the outside, for instance through a laparoscope.

The hormone tests seek to measure the abnormal amounts of hormones, especially luteinizing hormone, produced in excess by the ovarian tissue (stroma) surrounding the follicles. If previous tests have suggested that ovarian function is doubtful, a biopsy (small fragment of tissue taken for diagnostic purposes) is occasionally taken to confirm certain conditions, e.g., premature menopause, in which the ovary runs out of eggs too early in life.

A careful search is made for the presence of brown or black spots suggestive of endometriosis. This condition, which I described in the last chapter, is a prime cause of infertility, although, fortunately, it can now be treated easily in the majority of cases (see p. 74).

During laparoscopy the doctor will be especially interested in the Fallopian tubes. Their overall appearance may suggest previous infection (salpingitis). Salpingitis may be shown by the presence of adhesions and an abnormal appearance of the covering layer of the tube. Adhesions can cause infertility by binding down the tube, restricting its mobility and preventing it from picking up the ovum released by the ovary. Infection can also cause infertility by destroying the delicate lining of the tube, preventing the ovum from passing into the uterus.

Adhesions in the pelvis or abdomen also form to a greater or lesser extent after any type of surgery, especially operations in the pelvis. The condition of ectopic pregnancy, for example, in which a tiny fetus and placenta become attached and start to develop in the Fallopian tube instead of in the uterus, almost always requires an operation, and the affected part of the tube is usually removed. It is usually impossible for ova to pass through the portion of the tube remaining, and occasionally subsequent adhesions bind down the other tube, inhibiting its ability to transport ova and further impairing fertility. The doctor will therefore spend some time examining the tubes closely to make sure they are fully mobile (occasionally by passing a thin probe into the abdomen to move the tubes about directly).

Testing for tubal patency

The next step is to see whether the tubes are open (patent) along their entire length. This can be shown by passing a dark-coloured water-soluble dye up the intrauterine tube, thus filling the uterus with dye. If the tubes are open, the dye will pass along them and spill into the abdominal cavity at the ends. The passage of the dye along the inside of the tube can be seen through the laparoscope, since the outside of the tube will be slightly darkened by the dye. If the tube is blocked, the site of the obstruction can often be located. If the tube is completely blocked, or blocked near its junction with the uterus, no dye will pass. When injecting the dye a gentle pressure only is applied in order not to disturb the delicate inner lining of the tube.

Curettage

After the dye has been passed and tubal function assessed, a curettage of the uterus may be performed. This allows the doctor to take a sample of the lining of the uterus (endometrial biopsy). As we saw on p. 41, some doctors take an endometrial biopsy at the time of the physical examination earlier on in the investigations to check whether ovulation has occurred. If there is still any doubt at laparoscopy about whether the woman is ovulating an endometrial biopsy can settle the issue.

The intrauterine tube used to carry the dye is removed and a small sharp-edged spoonlike instrument—a curette—is inserted into the uterine cavity. With a few firm strokes of the curette inside the uterus, tissue from the endometrium is removed for later analysis. In particular, the appearance of the endometrial tissue can suggest that ovulation has occurred (which is why this examination is usually performed in the second half of the menstrual cycle). Biopsies can also be sent to the laboratory for the detection of infections such as tuberculosis, an occasional cause of infertility.

Completing laparoscopy

The doctor will always make every effort to ensure that women are not pregnant at the time of these examinations and procedures; as I mentioned earlier, women frequently become pregnant early on during investigations in the reassuring knowledge that something is being done. It would be a disaster to destroy a long-awaited pregnancy by performing a curettage and passing dye before making certain that the woman is not pregnant at the time.

The whole procedure of laparoscopy, passing dye and curettage is normally completed within half an hour, is relatively safe, and yields a great deal of information about the state of the gynaecological organs. A surgeon is able to assess whether operations such as surgery to repair the Fallopian tubes, removal of fibroids, or removal of adhesions by lysis (the surgical term meaning to cut or remove adhesions to free bound down organs), are feasible so that he or she can discuss the pros and cons comprehensively with the couple concerned beforehand. Sometimes the surgeon will perform the laparoscopy by itself and then, after discussion, arrange to do the tubal surgery at a later date. A laparoscopy and dye takes about 20 minutes—tubal surgery may take two hours and this amount of operating theatre time will need to be booked ahead. In special circumstances the surgeon will arrange to perform the laparoscopy and dye with a view to proceeding to tubal surgery and carry this out under the same anaesthetic. The surgeon will make the proposed arrangements quite clear to the woman before the operation, that is, whether it is to be laparoscopy and dye by itself or laparoscopy, dye and an option to proceed to tubal surgery if necessary.

On removing the laparoscope the gas is expelled from the abdomen and a suture or two placed in the small incision. The patient can leave hospital quite soon after the operation in most cases. Many women return home after three to six hours' observation following laparoscopy, although some stay in the hospital overnight. Most women are walking about after a few hours. Complaints afterwards are few but may include those resulting from the anaesthesia (sore throat, general muscle aches, nausea) and those caused by the laparoscope—painful umbilicus, menstrual cramps, vaginal bleeding, etc. If any gas remains in the abdomen it is usually absorbed slowly into the bloodstream. Occasionally, however, it will rise to the top of the abdomen and irritate the diaphragm. Since the diaphragm is supplied by sensory nerves which also supply the skin over the tip of the shoulder, pain from such diaphragmatic irritations is referred to (i.e., felt in) the shoulder—usually passing within a day or two.

I said a few moments ago that laparoscopy is a relatively safe procedure; however, as it is usually performed under a general anaesthetic, the patient is subject to the small but ever-present risks that this carries. Although it is unlikely that problems will arise, they can occur, and that is why preliminary tests must be completed and the husband must be excluded as a possible cause of infertility before laparoscopy is performed.

7

Miscarriage

Miscarriage and infertility

This chapter is included in a book about infertility with reservation. Infertility is essentially an inability to conceive, whereas miscarriage can occur only after conception. However, a miscarried embryo or fetus is lost from the womb before it is viable (able to exist independently outside its mother's body) and the result is as in infertility—an empty cot. In addition, many women who have had troubles with miscarriage are nowadays investigated and advised in infertility clinics.

It has been my intention throughout this book to avoid lengthy discourses on any particular area of infertility without relating it to the practical situation of a couple being investigated in an average clinic. However, in dealing with miscarriage I feel obliged to depart from this and wish to explain briefly the different types of miscarriage, what is thought to happen, how miscarriage is investigated and treated, and hope that you will recognize features which are familiar to your particular situation.

First and foremost, I should explain the multitude of different terms pertaining to miscarriage. Doctors tend to use them, sometimes offhandedly, as if everyone knows their exact meaning, and this can cause a great deal of confusion, and even distress. It is sometimes difficult for a doctor, who may be working in a busy obstetric and gynaecological unit where several miscarriages are dealt with every day, to remember that a couple may not know what a miscarriage is, what it implies and what can be done about it. When I think back to the days before I was a medical student (not all that long ago), I suppose I had a vague idea of what a miscarriage meant, i.e., simply that the woman lost the baby before it was ready to be born. Like most people, I suppose, some of my impressions derived from films, where every miscarriage seemed to start off with a riding or car accident, or with the husband hitting his pregnant wife, and the actual miscarriage happened up in the bedroom (out of sight of the camera) and ended with the doctor walking slowly down the stairs and shaking his head.

Let me say immediately that doctors do not usually use the term miscarriage—they say 'abortion'. However, since the term abortion is used by most people to mean a deliberately induced termination of pregnancy rather than the accidental loss of a fetus, I shall use the term miscarriage to prevent confusion. In the United Kingdom a fetus is not considered viable if born before 28 weeks of gestation. Since many special care units are able to save some babies younger than 28 weeks nowadays this arbitrary age limit is under review. However, in plain terms, if the mother loses her pregnancy before 28 weeks and the baby is unable to live outside her womb, she has miscarried, whether the baby is alive or dead when it passes out of the womb. If the baby is born dead after 28 weeks it is called a stillbirth; if it is born alive before term the birth is said to be premature.

Terminology

Most miscarriages, whether early or late, follow or are accompanied by bleeding from the uterus through the vagina. Sometimes little blood is lost, sometimes a dangerously large amount. Bleeding in pregnancy before 28 weeks heralds a possible miscarriage and is therefore referred to as a 'threatened abortion' (miscarriage). In a threatened miscarriage the woman is usually given bed rest, not necessarily in hospital, in the hope that the bleeding will settle down and eventually stop. If, however, the cervix (neck of the womb) opens up (this is frequently associated with uterine contractions—mini-labour pains) the conceptus (fetus and placenta) will subsequently be passed out. At this stage doctors speak of an 'inevitable abortion'. If the fetus and placenta along with its membranes all pass out of the uterus completely, the term used is 'complete abortion', and if any bits and pieces remain inside the uterus it is called an 'incomplete abortion'. All fairly logical, I think you will agree.

Danger of infection   If either the dead fetus or the placenta remain inside the uterus after miscarriage, there is a serious risk of that essentially dead tissue becoming infected. Any such remnants are usually scraped out, with the woman under general anaesthetic, by gentle curettage of the womb—usually referred to as an ERPC (evacuation of retained products of conception). This is like an ordinary 'D and C' (dilatation of the cervix and curettage of the uterus) and usually is performed within several hours of an incomplete miscarriage occurring. The dilatation is often unnecessary as the cervix will be open already, and the curettage is performed gently so as not to perforate the soft muscle of the uterus. Strict precautions are observed to prevent the introduction of infection. If the woman's temperature remains normal, and there is no vaginal bleeding afterwards, she is usually released from hospital after a day or so. But if infection intervenes the term 'septic abortion' is applied. Big doses of antibiotics are given by injection, and as soon as the worst of the infection is under control, an ERPC is performed to remove the infected material. Before the days of antibiotics, septic abortions were frequently fatal and even now occasionally a woman's life may be lost if the treatment is inadequate or delayed.

One particular type of infection, caused by bacteria called clostridia, produces 'gas gangrene' with the release of toxins into the blood which may kill within a few hours; doctors may be unable to prevent death despite intensive recovery procedures. Every effort, therefore, is made to prevent a woman who has miscarried from getting an infection. Thankfully in modern times very few women do, and nearly all women who miscarry have nothing to fear from infection. However, when infection intervenes but does not kill, there is a big danger of subsequent infertility. As you can imagine, virulent infection inside the womb is bound to affect the Fallopian tubes to a greater or lesser extent, and tubal blockage and damage may result, as it may from other types of infection discussed previously. Under these circumstances the woman's subsequent fertility may be impaired. In the vast majority of women fertility is *not* impaired after miscarriage—contrary to the impression given by those Hollywood movies.

This brings me to the subject of induced, or therapeutic, abortion. An abortion (miscarriage) which occurs without provocation is termed 'spontaneous'. The majority of miscarriages, for reasons which will become apparent later, do occur out of the blue—not after motor accidents, not after emotional upsets, not after any specific event—they just happen. Of course, it is true that special events of this kind may very occasionally precipitate a miscarriage, particularly trauma to the abdomen or a high fever during pregnancy. We also know that there is a high risk of miscarriage if abdominal operations (for example, to remove an ovarian cyst) are performed during middle to late pregnancy; but don't get the idea that miscarriage is always preceded by some special event. Miscarriage is common and may well coincide with some circumstance, such as an emotional upset; people like to ascribe a cause to miscarriage whereas in most cases no direct stimulus exists.

Induced (therapeutic) abortion

However, throughout human history women have found themselves undesirably pregnant, and miscarriage procured by interference inside the uterus, or by taking noxious drugs (abortifacients), is, and has been, a feature of nearly every society, civilized or uncivilized. Deliberately procured miscarriage is known as 'induced abortion'. Although it has frequently been outlawed (in Denmark during the last century abortionists and aborted women were decapitated and their heads placed on a pole for all to see), in many countries today, of course, induced abortion is performed within the confines of the law, in approved medical institutions, for defined reasons. In this case it is often referred to as 'therapeutic abortion'. The operation may be performed because the mother would be in danger if the pregnancy continued, or there may be a very high risk that the baby will be born deformed, e.g., if the mother has contracted rubella (German measles) in the first few months of pregnancy. Induced abortion (which is often known medically as a TOP—termination of pregnancy), even when performed in experienced medical centres, can on occasion be followed by infection which may result in infertility if not properly treated.

Causes of miscarriage   At the risk of boring you let me emphasize again just how common miscarriage is. About one pregnancy in every five or six ends in miscarriage in the United Kingdom. When you consider how many pregnancies there are every year, even in those Western countries with zero population growth, you can appreciate that an enormous number of miscarriages must take place. It is known that a large proportion of miscarriages (estimated at between 40 and 60 per cent) occur because there is something wrong with the fetus—frequently a chromosomal abnormality. The arrangement of chromosomes in the fertilized ovum is often incompatible with viability—or, in plain English, the pregnancy is defective, and the quicker it is passed out of the mother's body the better.

In some miscarriages the fetus completely fails to develop and an empty sac is passed. This is referred to as a 'blighted ovum', or 'missed abortion'—terms of which I and many others are not particularly fond, as they imply some disease process is at work. In many cases there has again been a mistake in the chromosomal construction, the plans are doomed from the start, and miscarriage in this event can be thought of as a quality control procedure.

Another factor causing miscarriage is the failure of the embryo, which may be quite normal, to implant itself properly in the lining of the uterus; or it may implant in a position which makes miscarriage likely, e.g. very low down in the uterus. This may be a result of hormonal failure. Hormone levels may have been insufficient to prepare the lining of the uterus to receive and sustain the embryo properly. The pregnancy is supported initially by hormones produced by the corpus luteum in the ovary, but in early pregnancy production of these hormones is handed over to the developing placenta. It is thought that if this hand-over of hormone production is ill-timed or inadequate, a drop in hormone levels results and is followed by miscarriage. This theory is not without defects, but it explains the occasional practice of giving hormones (usually of the progesterone type) to women with threatened miscarriage of whatever cause.

An abnormally shaped uterus may account for miscarriage. If this is the case, the miscarriage often occurs somewhat later in the pregnancy than those due to chromosomal abnormalities; the early embryo implants well but the growing fetus is not retained in the abnormal uterus. Corrective operations are usually offered, following HSGs and other investigations, if a misshapen womb is thought to be the prime cause of recurrent miscarriage (see p. 121).

In rare cases miscarriage is possibly attributable to severe diseases of the mother. Non-infective causes, such as kidney problems and very high blood pressure, have been suggested. However, on the whole, maternal diseases causing miscarriage are likely to be infective. A variety of infections have been implicated, including rubella (German measles), poliomyelitis, and other viral infections, T-mycoplasma (an organism between a virus and a bacterium), and certain bacterial infections such as tuberculosis, syphilis, toxoplasmosis, brucellosis, listeriosis (although the last two may only affect animals), and, in areas where the disease is endemic, malaria. Let me stress that these are uncommon causes, but where they are suspected, the doctor will investigate and treat the woman appropriately.

Dietary factors have also been suggested as a cause of miscarriage; the evidence has not been conclusive, but various vitamin deficiencies have been investigated, and folic-acid deficiency in particular. A possible explanation for a very small number of miscarriages is that the mother rejects the fetus. A gross example of this is rhesus iso-immunization, in which a sensitized rhesus-negative mother 'attacks' a rhesus-positive fetus in the uterus, leading in some cases to fetal death and miscarriage. Fetal tissue is essentially foreign to the mother, but is not normally rejected by the mother's immunological processes. Doctors do not understand completely why the fetus enjoys this immunological protection, but it is not difficult to understand that if this protective mechanism breaks down the fetus would then be rejected and subsequently miscarry. Interesting research is going on in London at present looking for a possible link between miscarriage and antibodies raised by the father's bloodstream.

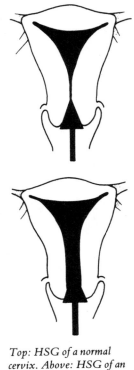

Top: HSG of a normal cervix. Above: HSG of an incompetent cervix, showing the classic funnel shape.

Miscarriage later on in the pregnancy is usually a problem of accommodation. In the first three months (trimester) of pregnancy the rise in hormone levels stimulates the growth of the uterus, and this increase in size is greater than the growth of the conceptus (fetus, membranes, placenta, amniotic fluid, etc.). However, at three months the conceptus fills the womb and as it enlarges rapidly, a concomitant growth of the uterus is required. The placenta is strongly attached to the wall of the uterus. As the fetus grows its weight is transmitted to the cervix. If the cervix is weak (incompetent) and starts to open up, there is a danger that a miscarriage will occur through simple mechanical failure. The sort of factors which can lead to a degree of cervical incompetence in some cases (but by no means all) are weakening through previous deliveries of babies, late therapeutic abortions where the opening in the cervix (os) has been severely stretched, and operations on the cervix (e.g., cone biopsy) for early cancers. Sometimes a potentially incompetent cervix may be discovered early on by vaginal examination or be anticipated following hysterosalpingograms before the pregnancy, where a funnel-shaped appearance of the cervical canal will be seen. Women who have had surgery to the cervix, for example a cone biopsy, tend to be examined more frequently than usual during pregnancy, and any dilatation of the cervix can be dealt with early on.

Treatment of cervical incompetence

Let me first deal with cervical incompetence causing relatively late miscarriage. The cervix usually opens up quite painlessly and at first the membranes bulge through the os, then they rupture, the fluid is lost, the womb contracts rhythmically and the conceptus is expelled.

The commonest way to deal with this problem is to insert a purse-string suture (frequently a strong tape) around the neck of the womb beneath its surface, and tie a knot. This type of cervical encirclage is often referred to as a 'Shirodkar' after the surgeon who pioneered it. The suture stops the cervix from opening up. The operation is performed under general anaesthetic (i.e., fully asleep) at about the fourteenth week of pregnancy, after the chance of an early miscarriage before 12 weeks has passed, but before the baby and its afterbirth (placenta) have become

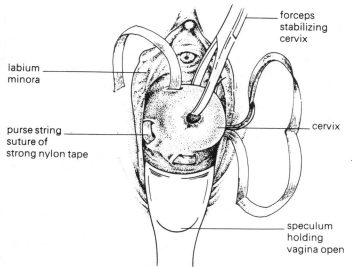

forceps
stabilizing
cervix

labium
minora

purse string
suture of
strong nylon tape

cervix

speculum
holding
vagina open

*An incompetent cervix is
sutured with strong nylon
tape (shown actual size)
which is pulled tight and
fastened. This operation is
done under general
anaesthetic at about 14–16
weeks of pregnancy. The
suture causes no subsequent
discomfort, but the woman
will be monitored carefully
for the possibility of infection.*

heavy enough to push the incompetent cervix open.

Occasionally as the pregnancy progresses the suture cuts loose and a second or even a third suture needs to be inserted. In most women the suture is removed at about 38 weeks of pregnancy, or earlier if labour commences, and the birth proceeds normally. In some women the suture is left in place and the baby is delivered by planned Caesarean section.

Treating early miscarriage

Matters are not so straightforward in the case of early miscarriage. Since many women will have at least one miscarriage during their lives, few doctors will be perturbed by the case of a woman who has had one or even two miscarriages at say 12 weeks' gestation. Recurrent or habitual miscarriage is defined as three or more consecutive miscarriages. Women who have had recurrent miscarriages usually want to be told why, but in many cases their doctor will be unable to say. Examination of the miscarried fetus under the microscope may indicate possible chromosomal or other congenital problems, but in all too many women no definite cause is found. However, an attempt is usually made to rule out as many causes as possible, and blood tests are taken for toxoplasma, syphilis, T-mycoplasma, iso-antibodies, diabetes, thyroid function, etc. Hysterosalpingograms are indicated if there is a suspicion of uterine abnormality or cervical incompetence. Any signs of infection or raised levels of antibodies in the bloodstream will be followed up with the appropriate treatment.

If hormone deficiences are suspected there is in most cases little that can be done, as giving the mother hormones has not proved to help a great deal. This implies that she is short of hormones because the placenta is failing and that the drop in hormones may well be a side-effect rather than a prime cause of the problem. In the past oestrogens have been administered in early pregnancy, but this has had the disastrous side-effect of stimulating vaginal cancers in the female offspring in a few cases.

Threatened miscarriage is usually dealt with by bed rest, often in hospital, in the hope that the bleeding will settle down. During these anxious days of waiting the woman frequently pleads for or demands something more active in the way of treatment to save her pregnancy, and hormones, such as progestogens, are frequently given primarily to reassure her, as the doctor will probably doubt their efficacy.

As can be imagined, the psychological support of a woman with a threatened or actual miscarriage by doctors, nurses, family and friends is a very important part of caring for her. Much reassurance must be offered and any misplaced feelings of guilt overcome. But it is often difficult to reassure a woman who has had five or six miscarriages for which no cause can be found with a few platitudes about how frequent an occurrence miscarriage is.

During the period of bed rest pregnancy tests are made repeatedly, usually by measuring levels of the hormone HCG (human chorionic gonadotrophin) in the urine or blood. If the bleeding persists or gets worse, bits of conceptus are passed out and a positive pregnancy test may become negative; then an ERPC can be performed as the fetus would appear to have died. This may occur over a few days.

Ultrasound scans (using high-frequency sound waves) of these early pregnancies can often indicate accurately whether the fetus is still alive, and therefore avoid two or three unnecessary and anxious days in hospital. Often when the woman has had some bleeding she is very anxious and may not be sure if she has passed any 'bits and pieces' likely to be parts of the conceptus. An immediate ultrasound scan can be performed to see what is going on in the uterus. If no movement can be detected and only a few small disarranged pieces of conceptus can be seen, the woman has had an incomplete miscarriage. She can have an ERPC without delay and be discharged soon—thus avoiding several anxious days of misery.

Every now and then the amount of bleeding at miscarriage is so heavy that the woman will require blood transfusion. When her condition becomes stable an ERPC can be performed and the uterus encouraged to contract and stop bleeding by the use of certain drugs (such as those derived from the ergot alkaloids which cause vigorous uterine contractions, squeezing bleeding vessels closed).

In conclusion, remember that miscarriage is common and many women will have at least one in their lives. It does not necessarily suggest trouble lies ahead for subsequent pregnancies. In many cases it is simply a case of quality control to eliminate an imperfect conceptus. The cause and possible treatment for recurrent or habitual miscarriages are rather obscure and much research throughout the world is geared to this problem. Some interesting research in London is being conducted into the role of the immune system in recurrent miscarriage. Some evidence suggests that certain women might be immunized with substances from their partners' blood components which may prevent subsequent miscarriage. Whereas this approach is interesting and welcome, it is unlikely that large numbers of women who miscarry will benefit from the immune system treatment methods now being investigated.

8

Induction of ovulation

Disorders of ovulation account for the failure to conceive in about 10 to 15 per cent of infertile couples. Fortunately, however, the treatment of women who fail to ovulate is one of the most successful areas of infertility therapy, and the prospects for most of these 'anovulatory' women are good. In recent years several drugs to induce ovulation by stimulating the ovaries have become available—the so-called 'fertility drugs'. Contrary to the impression one gains from reading newspaper stories of women who give birth to five or more babies after fertility treatment, the risks of multiple births are quite low. In fact there are two stages of drug treatment, and the second stage is only begun if the woman fails to respond to the first. It is in this second, more powerful treatment stage that the risks of multiple ovulation increase more sharply, but here careful monitoring of the patient by the medical team can minimize this danger.

Before going into all this in more detail I shall briefly recap the course of the investigations leading up to the induction of ovulation, beginning with how the doctor has arrived at the knowledge that the woman is not ovulating.

The story so far
If a woman is not menstruating at all then it is extremely unlikely that she is ovulating (producing a ripe ovum ready for fertilization). There is one general exception to this rule—the woman who has just stopped breast feeding a baby. She may ovulate in the period after childbirth without a normal menstrual bleed following. However,

for practical purposes, a woman who is not having regular periods is probably not ovulating. Similarly, a woman with scanty or very irregular periods *may* not be ovulating properly. The converse, however, is not necessarily true. It is known that a surprisingly high proportion of women who are not ovulating still have regular menstrual cycles of normal timing and duration. Clearly, the presence of bleeding is not enough to establish that ovulation is taking place.

Temperature charts are a good guide to whether or not a woman is ovulating: this has been demonstrated by studies which show that the typical 'biphasic' records correlate very closely with hormonal evidence of ovulation. Besides the temperature charts, other associated signs help confirm that ovulation is taking place, e.g., the intermenstrual pain of ovulation (mittelschmerz), changes in the amount of cervical mucus in the vagina in the second half of the cycle, a feeling of bloating due to water retention, breast tenderness and/or swelling, mood changes, and pain with the periods (dysmenorrhoea). These signs do not usually occur unless ovulation is taking place.

The doctor will usually check that ovulation has occurred by measuring the level of progesterone hormone in the blood during the second half of the cycle—a blood sample is usually taken on or around day 21 of the menstrual cycle (counting the first day of menstrual bleeding as day 1), and if the woman has ovulated the progesterone level should be substantially raised.

Primary and secondary amenorrhoea

Having got this far, the doctor knows that the woman is not ovulating at all; let us assume that she has no menstrual periods either. What will the next move be? Well, in those unusual cases where the woman has never menstruated in her life (primary amenorrhoea) the doctor will spend time excluding chromosomal disorders, the rare problems with the sex organs and sex hormones, and problems with the adrenal and pituitary glands, and the ovaries. He will, of course, treat any condition found as appropriate, and, if necessary, induce ovulation with fertility drugs. I have deliberately skimmed over the surface of primary amenorrhoea as this complex subject is beyond the scope of this book, and most of these women are usually investigated before they seek help for infertility.

So, the doctor in infertility work will be mainly faced with secondary amenorrhoea (i.e., the woman did have periods at one time, but they have since stopped). The cessation of periods can be a symptom of any one of a long list of problems and disorders I have mentioned, and I will cover only the major ones in more detail. In many women the cause of the amenorrhoea may not be found, but treatment can still be successful. Of course, where a cause is found, it must be corrected if possible.

The causes of failure of ovulation

Basically, the requirements for normal ovulation and menstruation are a normal uterus and ovaries, and the release of hormones from the pituitary gland, in appropriate quantities, to stimulate the ovaries. The amenorrhoea may result from faults in any of these: the uterus may be misshapen or damaged by infection; the ovary may be unresponsive because of polycystic disease or premature menopause; finally, and most frequently, the fault may lie in the pituitary gland or its 'boss' the hypothalamus, which is situated directly above it in the brain.

Pituitary gland/hypothalamic causes of amenorrhoea include emotional upsets—travel abroad, a change of job or lifestyle, important examinations; in such cases menstruation usually returns to normal spontaneously once the change of circumstance or anxiety has passed. Also included in this category are women whose weight has fallen below their menstruating norm, and women whose periods stop when oral contraceptives are discontinued (post-pill amenorrhoea). Women with more generalized diseases (e.g., depressive states, diabetes mellitus, overactive thyroid, or any severe debilitating illness) can also have amenorrhoea or scanty anovulatory menstrual periods. Where the adrenal gland secretes more hormones than it should (Cushing's syndrome or adrenal hyperplasia), ovulation may be inhibited. In unusual cases the pituitary gland itself may not be working too well.

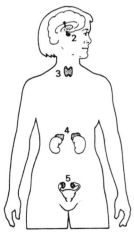

Endocrinal glands producing the hormones which influence female fertility.
1 Hypothalamus 2 Pituitary
3 Thyroid 4 Adrenal glands
5 Ovaries

Another pituitary cause of amenorrhoea, which we have already discussed, is raised levels of prolactin hormone in the blood (this may well result in a discharge from the breast as well as ovulation problems); this will be treated with the drug bromocriptine, and occasionally with other fertility drugs as well.

Tests will be done to investigate the cause of the problem—a hysterosalpingogram for possible uterine abnormalities, laparoscopy and ovarian biopsy (taking a small piece of ovary for examination) for possible ovarian problems, and a variety of blood tests to detect pituitary and hypothalamic defects. The doctor will choose the appropriate test depending on the patient's history and clinical examination.

Let us deal with several special causes of amenorrhoea. Firstly, premature menopause. Most women begin the menopause (the change of life, or normal cessation of periods) at around the same age (50 years in Western Europe). The ovaries simply stop producing ripe eggs. They also stop producing certain hormones, which may lead to other symptoms, e.g., hot flushes, but that is another story. The pituitary gland then produces larger amounts of follicle-stimulating hormone (FSH), but the ovaries remain unresponsive and do not produce an ovum. In a few unfortunate women this can happen earlier on in life, and when the menopause occurs before the age of 35 years it is termed premature. The diagnosis is aided by ovarian biopsy and the finding of elevated levels of FSH in the blood, but, regrettably, little or nothing can be done to help women who wish to conceive after a premature menopause. Very rarely the condition may occur in teenagers. The causes are not entirely known, but may be associated with the failure of other endocrine glands (adrenal, thyroid, pancreas), possible due to an immunity to one's own tissue (autoimmunity). Premature menopause may also occur in women with certain chromosomal abnormalities, e.g., Turner's syndrome.

Special causes of amenorrhoea

Polycystic ovaries may also account for anovulatory cycles. In this condition the ovaries are slightly enlarged and contain numerous little cysts. The diagnosis is made by ultrasound scanning of the ovaries (to look at their internal structure) and by measuring blood hormone levels—FSH and LH (see p. 107 later in this chapter). It is also occasionally made by removing a wedge of tissue from each ovary at operation. This technique is known as

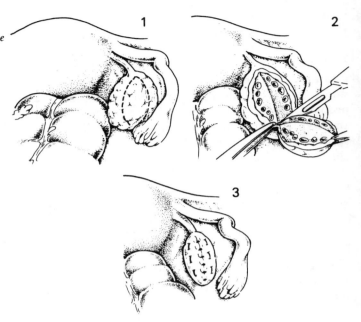

If a polycystic ovary is diagnosed by laparoscopy (see p. 87), the cysts may be removed in an operation known as wedge resection. 1 Sight of incision 2 Wedge of cystic ovary removed 3 Ovary is repaired.

wedge resection (see above).

Women with post-pill amenorrhoea (absence of periods after discontinuing oral contraceptives) and other women with amenorrhoea of unknown cause are usually treated with fertility drugs to induce ovulation.

The progesterone challenge

The doctor usually starts treatment of a non-ovulating woman who has no menstrual bleeding by creating an artificial period from which future fertility drug treatment can be dated. Sex hormones, frequently a synthetic progestogen similar to natural progesterone, are given in tablet form, for say 5 days (alternatively, a single injection of progesterone may be given); a withdrawal menstrual bleed usually follows within a week. The first day of bleeding can then be counted as day 1 of the artificial cycle and further treatment measured from there. As well as producing a starting base the period produced by this 'progesterone challenge' gives an indication that the uterus and its lining (endometrium) is responding reasonably well to the presence of the hormone. In women where the uterus has been severely damaged by infection, for example, the response to the challenge will be negative—

no period will ensue, and further investigations are required.

Switching on ovulation

We now have a woman who has a menstrual period but is not ovulating. The discussion which follows also applies to those women who have been having menstrual periods of some sort but were not ovulating. What is required is a drug which will 'switch on' the pituitary gland and cause it to produce the hormones necessary to stimulate the ovaries into producing a ripe ovum.

The drug frequently chosen to do that is clomiphene citrate; more recently tamoxifen has come into use. Although the mechanism by which clomiphene acts is not completely clear, we have known since 1964 that it reduces the uptake of oestrogen by the pituitary gland and hypothalamus, and the pituitary subsequently releases gonadotrophin hormones (luteinizing hormone, follicle-stimulating hormone) to stimulate the ovaries. The fertility drugs are thus acting on the body's hormonal feedback system, by which the pituitary and hypoth-alamus monitor the levels of hormones in the blood and release more hormones as necessary.

Their action is, in fact, the very reverse of the action of the oral contraceptive pill: the pill introduces extra oestrogens into the body, which has the effect of switching off the release of gonadotrophins from the pituitary. The fertility drugs, on the other hand, are 'anti-oestrogens'. By reducing the pituitary's sensitivity to oestrogen, they are in effect shouting at the lazy pituitary gland that not enough hormones have been secreted recently and not enough ova have been released by the ovaries. There is some evidence that clomiphene also has a direct effect on the ovaries, but the simplest way to regard clomiphene and tamoxifen is as anti-oestrogens which stimulate the pituitary into action to start the cycle off.

Administering clomiphene

There may be some variation in the dose, duration and timing of clomiphene administration from doctor to doctor, but the underlying principle remains the same. To give an example, one tablet (50 mg) per day is given on days 2 to 6, or days 5 to 10. If after one month menstruation has not occurred, or a pregnancy has not been produced (this is a very real possibility—I know of several women who have conceived after just one course of tablets), the dose can be doubled (100 mg) and trebled subsequently if necessary. The doctor watches for evidence of ovulation using temperature charts and day 21 serum progesterone blood tests (see p. 72), and if ovulation does occur clomiphene is continued cyclically at the appropriate dose level, and the couple are encouraged to have intercourse at the appropriate time in the cycle.

In these relatively small doses and short courses of treatment overstimulation of the ovaries is unusual, but some doctors will want to check by vaginal examination that the ovaries are not enlarged before each course of clomiphene. If enlargement is detected treatment is suspended until the ovarian swelling settles down (this usually takes about a month). Side effects of this drug are not common but 5–10 per cent of women have reported occasional hot flushes, similar to those experienced by menopausal women, while taking clomiphene and for a few days after. However, the same patient may not experience these symptoms in all treatment cycles and hardly any women are completely unable to take this effective treatment.

Effective treatment it is indeed—it produces ovulation in about three-quarters of patients with functional and secondary amenorrhoea (especially 'post-pill' amenorrhoea) and with the polycystic ovary syndrome. About a quarter of patients with primary amenorrhoea will also ovulate. Pregnancy, however, is the ultimate yardstick by which to judge the effectiveness of treatment, and providing the woman is healthy and failure of ovulation is the only problem affecting fertility (i.e., the Fallopian tubes are not blocked and the male partner is not infertile) most doctors would expect a 50 per cent chance of pregnancy.

Direct stimulation of the ovaries

Women who have not ovulated after clomiphene or tamoxifen treatment may well be considered for treatment with gonadotrophins. This consists of injections of follicle-stimulating hormone (FSH) which will directly induce the ovary to produce a ripe ovum. The treatment is complex, expensive, needs careful monitoring of the woman, and carries an ever-present risk of overstimulating the ovaries; this can produce discomfort for the woman and involves a high chance of multiple births. Therapy with gonadotrophins is therefore carried out by doctors in experienced centres with access to rapid laboratory hormone measurements.

Before the woman embarks on treatment with gonadotrophins, the couple will have been fully investigated and causes of infertility other than ovulatory failure will have been ruled out. The majority of women who receive this treatment will have failed to conceive on clomiphene. No doctor would offer this treatment without a full discussion with the couple, as their immediate cooperation is essential. I will only give a brief outline of the treatment as the actual details of gonadotrophin administration can vary from one doctor to another.

Gonadotrophins can be extracted from pituitary glands taken from cadavers, in which case they are referred to as human pituitary gonadotrophin or HPG. As you can imagine, this is not a very abundant source, especially when you consider that each gland is about the size of a pea. But there is another, much more plentiful supply. As I have already mentioned, at the time of the menopause (change of life) the ovaries stop producing ova, but the pituitary gland is not content with this state of affairs and 'shouts' at the ovaries, hormonally speaking, in order to get them to produce an ovum. Thus for some time after the menopause the level of FSH (follicle-stimulating hormone) secreted into the bloodstream by the pituitary is very elevated. This high level of FSH is excreted from the woman's body in her urine. The urine of postmenopausal women is thus a rich source, from which human menopausal gonadotrophin (HMG) can be extracted. Pure FSH is now becoming available and may eventually replace HMG.

In addition a luteinizing hormone is required and the one most frequently chosen is human chorionic gonadotrophin (HCG) which is secreted in large amounts during pregnancy, again passing out of the body in the urine, and as such forms the basis of many pregnancy tests. Treatment with HMG or HPG is usually given in conjunction with HCG.

Basically, a series of injections is given and ovulation is stimulated. Careful measurements of hormone levels in the urine or blood are made to make sure that the ovaries do not become overstimulated. This problem can produce symptoms varying between mild enlargement of the ovaries, up to more severe cases of abdominal enlargement, with nausea, vomiting and diarrhoea. Multiple ovulation may well result, leading to multiple pregnancy.

Further evidence of response to treatment may also be given by observing the cervical mucus and examining the vaginal tissue to look for the effects of oestrogen. The doctor will increase the dose of HMG or HPG given until satisfied that ovulation has been induced (the dose required varies from woman to woman) but if overstimulation is suggested by the tests, the HCG injection usually necessary will not be given.

The treatment schedule

Let me give you an example of a popular treatment schedule. Three intramuscular injections of equal doses of HMG are given on three alternate days (days 1, 3, and 5). On day 2 a 24-hour urine collection or a blood sample is taken and the level of oestrogen is measured to record a baseline. This is repeated on day 4 and day 6, to check that overstimulation has not occurred (if it had the oestrogen levels in the 24-hour urine samples would be very high). On day 8 another measurement of oestrogen is made to provide an indication of the dosage of HMG required for subsequent courses if necessary. Also on day 8, if all is well and the oestrogen level indicates that the ovary contains a ripe ovum, ready for ovulation, and there is no overstimulation of the ovaries, an injection of HCG is given to induce ovulation, the couple are advised to have intercourse on that day and the following day, and fingers are crossed in the hope of a pregnancy. The ripening of the follicle and the release of the ovum can be monitored by having daily ultrasound scans to watch the follicle swell and then 'pop' when the egg is released. This also indicates when intercourse should take place.

If all this strikes you as rather complex then I have succeeded in giving an accurate picture. It is complex. It requires a good deal of cooperation between the woman and a doctor who really knows what he or she is doing.

However, the high success rate makes the treatment eminently worthwhile: a study in 1972 followed up 269 women—who between them received 856 courses of HMG treatment. Ovulation occurred 398 times (47 per cent) and there were 85 pregnancies (28 per cent). Hyperstimulation occurred in 42 cases (15 per cent). In another study two years earlier of 287 pregnancies which went to term, 230 (80 per cent) had single births, 43 (15 per cent) had twins and 14 (5 per cent) triplets, quads, or quins. These treatments are carried out as an outpatient, but if a woman lives a considerable distance from the treatment centre she may have to stay in accommodation nearby.

During the last decade or so a great many women who were infertile because they were unable to ovulate properly have conceived after the administration of fertility drugs. Treatment of ovulation is the most successful area of infertility work. Its success contrasts markedly with the less successful area of tubal surgery, which is discussed in the next chapter.

Induction of ovulation by LH/RH pump

A new system of inducing ovulation is currently being assessed in Britain for women who have not been able to ovulate with other treatments, especially those with polycystic ovary syndrome. A little reservoir and pump is strapped around the woman's waist with a tiny tube and needle introduced underneath the skin of the arm. The pump injects a little luteinizing hormone releasing substance (LH/RH) into the woman in the days following a period, in order to promote the development of a follicle and subsequent release of an egg.

The LH/RH pump is an exciting new development in the treatment of women who are unable to ovulate on their own. One distinct advantage the LH/RH pump has over the direct stimulation of the ovaries by injections of FSH, is that it usually stimulates only one follicle, thus avoiding the risk of stimulating four, five, six or even more, as can happen with uncontrolled FSH injections.

Wearing the pump and receiving treatment causes very little inconvenience indeed and no pain. Most women who are working outside the home can wear the pump happily and carry on with their jobs. Around the time of ovulation they will need to attend hospital as an outpatient

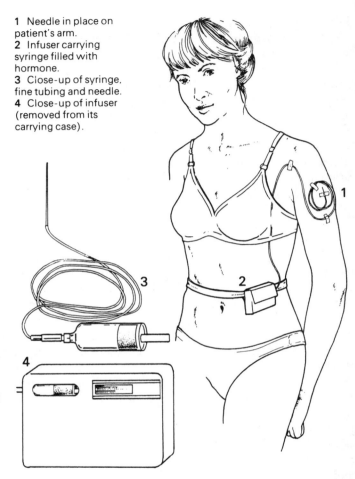

1 Needle in place on patient's arm.
2 Infuser carrying syringe filled with hormone.
3 Close-up of syringe, fine tubing and needle.
4 Close-up of infuser (removed from its carrying case).

The LH/RH pump enables intermittent and controlled doses of LH/RH to be injected to mimic the normal release from the hypothalamus in the brain. This new technique is more effective in avoiding over-stimulation of the ovaries.

to have serial ultrasound scans and any adjustments to their pump dose made.

Ovulation and endometriosis

There is another group of women who are not ovulating and who require further consideration—those whose failure to conceive is due to endometriosis. We have already discussed this condition as a possible cause of subfertility (see p. 74), and looked at the typical candidate and her symptoms—usually a woman in her 30s who experiences progressively more painful periods, occasional irregular bleeding, occasional deep pain on intercourse, and who has probably not conceived previously. The diagnosis might be confirmed at laparoscopy or laparotomy. If laparotomy is performed, the black spots of endometriosis in the pelvis might be excised (cut out) or cauterized (burned with electrical forceps).

Nevertheless, the mainstay of treatment as far as restoration of fertility is concerned is hormone manipulation. Just as the lining of the uterus (endometrium) is stimulated by hormones during the menstrual cycle, so the endometriotic spots enlarge and bleed under the same hormonal influence, hence some of the pain they cause. They also emit powerful hormones called prostaglandins, and this is believed to influence adversely ovulation and conception. The mechanism is far from fully understood. Treatment is geared to damping down the hormone stimulus which keeps these spots going, i.e., the menstrual cycle. This can be achieved by treatment with continuous hormones, for example by taking the combined oestrogen–progestogen contraceptive pill every day, without a break, for six to twelve months. This suppresses the periods completely and hopefully reduces or eradicates the endometriotic spots. It doesn't always work, but it is worth trying, since it has been shown that there is a much higher chance of conceiving if endometriosis can be cleared up and the black 'powder burn' areas of endometriosis scattered in the pelvis disappear.

Hormone treatment

Prolonged courses of continuous oestrogen–progestogen preparations in the fairly high doses used are not without possible side effects, as one would expect in this 'pseudo–pregnancy', including weight gain, water retention, headache, fatigue, and breast discomfort; breakthrough bleeding may occur in the early months of treatment.

An alternative and more recent drug used in the treatment of endometriosis is called danazol. Danazol is able to suppress the normal menstrual cycle by inhibiting the manufacture and/or release of pituitary gonadotrophins. This 'anti-gonadotrophin' therefore stops the stimulation of the ovaries by the pituitary gland, thereby suppressing the normal menstrual cycle; the endometrium does not develop and any endometriotic deposits begin to shrink. Danazol is now being used widely to treat endometriosis as an alternative to continuous oestrogen-progestogen treatment. It too has side effects: a moderate number of patients experience weight gain and mild breakthrough bleeding, and because the female hormones are suppressed, some anabolic (male-type) hormonal effects have been seen, such as the appearance of acne, mild facial hair growth and increased libido (a side effect which is not always as much fun as one might at first think). These side effects, if present, can be reduced by adjusting the doses of danazol used.

There does not seem to be much difference in the pregnancy rate achieved in women with infertility secondary to endometriosis, whether oestrogen-progestogen treatment or danazol is used. Both in Britain and in the United States, a pregnancy rate of over 50 per cent is the norm, depending on the severity of the endometriosis. Danazol, however, would appear to relieve dysmenorrhoea (painful periods) associated with endometriosis more rapidly than the oestrogen-progestogen treatment does. Treatment with danazol is more expensive than with oestrogen-progestogen.

In some cases surgery is recommended with or without tablet treatment. Scarring around the Fallopian tubes and ovaries may develop as a reaction to endometriosis, and this might interfere with the release and transport of ova. The scars might be removed surgically and areas of endometriosis cauterized at operation. In any event, if conception does not occur within a year of discontinuing danazol or oestrogen-progestogen treatment, a 'second-look' laparoscopy might be advised to determine whether the endometriosis is completely eradicated and that there is no residual scarring.

9

Corrective surgery

If a woman is ovulating satisfactorily, and her partner shows evidence of potential fertility, the remaining obstacles to fertility are principally mechanical. The more complicated investigative procedures described on pp. 79 and 83—the hysterosalpingogram and laparoscopy—may have shown up some of these problems. The Fallopian tubes may be blocked or immobile, being bound down by adhesions of scar tissue, or the doctor may suspect that the lining of the tubes is damaged. There may be some abnormality in the size, shape or position of the uterus. In this chapter we shall look at which of these problems are amenable to surgery, what the various operations entail, and what the chances of success are.

Let us turn first to the Fallopian tubes, since they are the most likely site of 'mechanical' failure. As mentioned before, tubal damage and blockage is likely to follow infections in the genital tract and pelvis, of whatever cause. When not obviously due to a particular problem, such as an infected appendix, a generalized infection involving the upper genital tract, especially the Fallopian tubes and ovaries, is usually referred to as 'Pelvic Inflammatory Disease' (PID). PID has several causes, mostly infection by bacteria. Whatever the cause the residual damage to the tubes may vary from minimal, in which case their normal function is often maintained, through moderate to severe damage and possible abscess formation. PID may be treated quickly by bed-rest and antibiotics in many women, but in some, treatment may be prolonged and it

The Fallopian tubes

may be months or even a year before the symptoms of tenderness settle down.

Tubal surgery is usually reserved for removing blocked segments of a tube and re-joining it. It is, of course, theoretically possible for the tubes to remain patent (open) and for the delicate tubal lining, so important for transporting the egg from ovary to uterus, to be damaged by infection. In practice, however, this is unlikely. The tubes have a very narrow bore and during infections this narrow lumen (space) is frequently blocked off for good. It has been suggested that in some lucky women these blocked tubes may regenerate well enough to open up and allow an ovum access to the womb.

Even if the tubes did remain open after the infection had passed, when they were seen by the doctor at laparoscopy or laparotomy they would show scar tissue and surrounding adhesions, clearly indicating that there had been an infection. In cases where there is a suspicion that the lining is damaged, it can be examined using a bifocal operating microscope, and an experienced doctor can distinguish between a normal healthy glandular lining and a flattened damaged lining, which is unlikely to sustain the fertilized ovum in its two- or three-day journey to the safety of the uterus.

However, the proof of the pudding is in the eating, and the proof of tube function is pregnancy. Every effort will have been made to ensure that the woman is ovulating properly, and if the tubes appear to be open, and reasonably free from adhesions, then there will be little call for corrective surgery. Unfortunately, in a sizeable proportion of women the Fallopian tubes are found to be blocked, or greatly mis-shapen, and bound down by adhesions. If the tubes have not been totally destroyed it is technically possible to perform surgery to open them up and release the adhesions. Note that I said *technically* possible. In practice, if the tubes are blocked, much or indeed all of their lining tends to be destroyed, and even if they can be opened up by surgery they remain function-less. It cannot be said too often that the tubes are not just little funnels down which the ova slide into the uterus. No indeed; the delicate lining nurtures and possibly nourishes the ovum, provides the site for fertilization, and after several days have passed, allows the little zygote produced access into the uterus. If it were a matter of a simple funnel, one could replace blocked Fallopian tubes with tubes made of plastic.

The mobility of the tube seems to be important too— we know that at the time of ovulation the finger-like projections at the end of the tubes (fimbriae) pass over the surface of the ovary and pick up the ovum upon its release from the follicle. It is not difficult, therefore, to imagine how considerable adhesions can bind down the surface of the ovary with fibrous bands, and how when the Fallopian tube is also pulled away by distorting adhesions this can result in infertility.

Cut those adhesions away, I hear you say, open up those tubes! Yes, this can be done. But the results obtained, even by the most expert of surgical teams, are often disappointing, especially when the tube lining is damaged.

The risks of tubal surgery

Tubal surgery requires cutting into and opening up the abdomen (laparotomy)—and an operating time of possibly one or more hours—with all the risks attendant upon the use of a general anaesthetic. This is usually followed by about two weeks in hospital and not a little post-operative discomfort. It is not a matter for rushing into without due advice and counselling with the facts on the table.

There is an added risk in Fallopian-tube surgery. If surgery restores tubal patency, but leaves residual damage causing a narrowing or partial blockage of the tube, there is a chance that a fertilized ovum could get stuck in the tube and begin to develop and grow there (ectopic pregnancy). Ectopic pregnancies will eventually cause heavy bleeding within the pelvis, necessitating an urgent operation to remove the pregnancy from the tube. Where the pregnancy is very small, it is occasionally possible to excise the developing embryo and repair the Fallopian tube or reimplant it into the uterus. However, in many cases most of the tube has to be removed—rendering the woman's chances of conceiving even less.

However, after discussing matters fully with the couple, with the findings of a laparoscopy and/or hysterosalpingogram at hand, a surgeon may well offer the woman an operation to restore tubal patency and mobility, but will

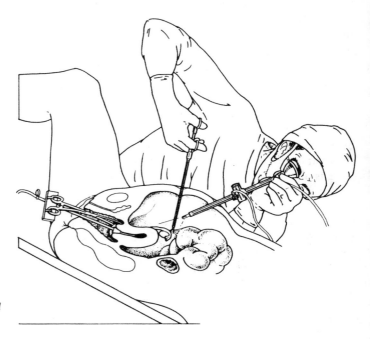

Cutting adhesions from the Fallopian tube and ovary, using microscissors observed through a laparoscope.

be quick to point out that the chances of producing a pregnancy are usually only a few per cent (though this depends on the extent of the damage), and that there is an enhanced risk of an ectopic pregnancy. However, where all other causes of infertility are ruled out many women are prepared to take the chance for the sake of the essentially very small hope of success.

What happens in tubal surgery

At operation any adhesions around the ovary, tubes and womb can be divided (cut), and full mobility is restored. This procedure is fairly straightforward, and if no other repair is required, there is a reasonable chance of conceiving afterwards—up to 40 per cent. If the ends of the tubes are blocked at the fimbriae, and there is not much damage to the rest of the tube, it is sometimes possible to open out the fimbriae again with gentle probing. If the fimbriae are destroyed cuts can be made into the blocked end of the tube (salpingostomy) to make an artificial wide opening. This procedure occasionally succeeds in producing a subsequent pregnancy. When the ends of the tubes are blocked, they become swollen and filled with fluid (hydrosalpinges) and this is severely damaging to their subsequent function. It must be said that if there are just a few adhesions which need separating, and the fimbriae can be straightened out undamaged from a recently blocked pair of tubes, then salpingostomy might well be successful. Such cases are unusual. Frequently, after substantial infection the tubes are ballooned out, like little sausages, with considerable damage and adhesions, placing the chances of conception into the realms of the miraculous.

If one or both of the tubes does not appear badly damaged, but it is known from laparoscopy and/or HSG studies that the mid-portion is blocked, the diseased segment can be cut out, the two ends joined, and a shortened, patent tube produced. This is a similar situation to the one the surgeon is faced with when reversing a sterilization; some of the problems of re-joining Fallopian tubes are discussed in detail on p. 128. But even when this technique is performed by the most skilful of surgeons, perhaps using microsurgical techniques, and patency of the tubes is confirmed by a subsequent HSG examination, this operation meets with only limited functional success, i.e., success as measured by pregnancies produced; and certainly the chance of an ectopic pregnancy is increased.

Tubal surgery does, however, meet with some success

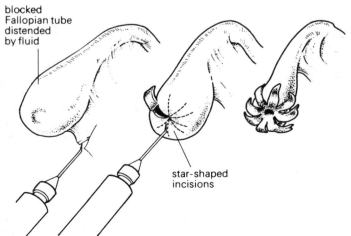

blocked
Fallopian tube
distended
by fluid

star-shaped
incisions

Blocked Fallopian tubes become distended with fluid (hydrosalpinges). Modern microsurgical techniques enable them to be opened (salpingostomy).

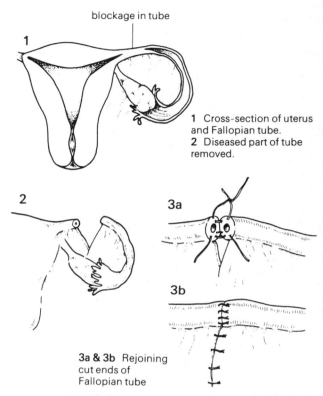

blockage in tube

1 Cross-section of uterus and Fallopian tube.
2 Diseased part of tube removed.

3a & 3b Rejoining cut ends of Fallopian tube

A blocked Fallopian tube can be repaired by cutting away the blocked portion and rejoining the patent ends.

when the tubes are blocked near to the point where they join the uterus (the cornua), providing the remainder of the tube looks healthy. In this operation the diseased tube is cut out and the new end of the tube reimplanted into the uterus. The muscle of the womb is cut during this procedure, which may weaken its performance during a subsequent labour, so Caesarean section is frequently advised if this operation has been performed.

To keep the tube open some surgeons leave little nylon strings inside the tube, going down into the uterus, as splints to be removed after healing has taken place. Other surgeons do not do this, believing that the splints may damage the delicate lining of the tube. Some surgeons give steroids (anti-inflammatory hormonal drugs) to the woman during and after the operation in order to decrease the amount of post-operative inflammation. The uterus and tubes may also be 'washed through' in the days following the operation (hydrotubation). All surgeons pay meticulous attention to decreasing the amount of bleeding at operation and keeping the chance of infection to an absolute minimum. If there is more than a drop or two of blood around, especially inside the Fallopian tube, then adhesions may be formed, ruining the whole attempt to restore tubal function. The value of steroids is not definitely known to be of help, but the idea of giving them seems sensible.

In the normal woman ovulation alternates each month between the two ovaries. In the past some surgeons would, on finding one diseased tube and one normal tube, remove the ovary from the diseased side to encourage ovulation to occur every month on the good side. This was often performed at operations to remove an ectopic pregnancy. The practice has largely been discontinued for several reasons, the main ones being, first, that it has been known for an ovum from one ovary to make its way into the tube on the *opposite* side and second, that no surgeon can be absolutely sure that function will never return to a damaged tube, however unlikely this may appear.

If both tubes appear so badly damaged as to be totally useless, but the uterus and ovaries seem reasonably normal, then the woman might be a suitable candidate for 'in vitro fertilization' (see Chapter 11). It must be emphasized that this procedure is still not very widely available, but it does offer hope to women for whom tubal surgery is useless or has failed.

Abnormalities of the uterus

A misshapen uterus may be thought to be a cause of infertility in a very few women. The problem with uterine abnormalities usually lies not so much in becoming pregnant as in holding the pregnancy inside. A small, underdeveloped (hypoplastic) uterus, for example, will be unable to carry a pregnancy. Unfortunately, nothing can be done to help women with a hypoplastic uterus; fortunately, they are very rare. It must be pointed out that many women with abnormally shaped wombs, of which a bicornuate (two-horned) uterus is one of the most common forms, have no trouble in conceiving or proceeding to term and delivery of a healthy baby. If recurrent miscarriage is a problem though, an operation to

Correcting abnormalities of the uterus

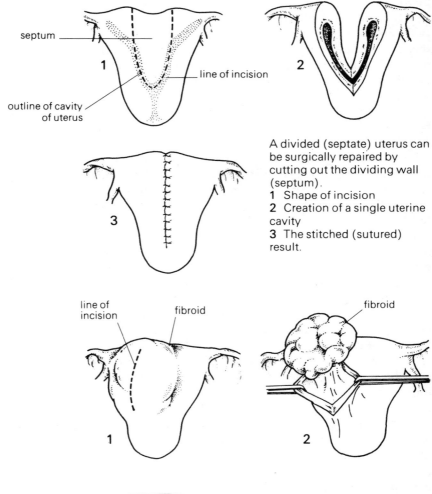

septum

line of incision

outline of cavity
of uterus

1

2

3

A divided (septate) uterus can
be surgically repaired by
cutting out the dividing wall
(septum).
1 Shape of incision
2 Creation of a single uterine
cavity
3 The stitched (sutured)
result.

line of
incision

fibroid

fibroid

1

2

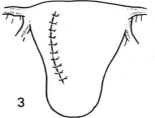

3

Fibroids can be 'shelled out'
of the uterus by an operation
known as myomectomy.

create a more normal uterine shape is usually offered. (See pp. 88–9.)

A womb distorted by multiple fibroids, which are benign tumours of the uterine muscle and occur to a greater or lesser extent in many women, may in a very few cases be thought to be the cause of a woman's infertility. The fibroids (or myomata) can be shelled out of the uterus in an operation known as myomectomy. But whereas they may account for some cases of infertility, they are more likely to be implicated in cases of recurrent miscarriage (see pp. 96–7).

Retroversion of the uterus

The round ligaments attached to the uterus, like the guy ropes of a tent, tend to keep it tilted forwards. This is known as anteversion. In some women the top of the uterus is angled forwards on the body of the womb—this is anteflexion. In about 20 per cent of women the womb is tilted backwards—retroversion.

In the past retroversion was thought to contribute to infertility and women with retroverted uteruses were offered an operation to pull the uterus forward by shortening the round ligaments. This procedure is nowadays much less popular as an aid to fertility. Two further points are worthy of mention in this connection. It is now thought that the position of the uterus, either retroverted or anteverted, is far less important than its mobility. If the uterus appears to be immobile on vaginal examination the doctor will suspect that it might be bound down by adhesions resulting from previous inflammation and infection. Thus *fixed* retroversion associated with infertility might need investigation and treatment.

The operation to correct retroversion might however be offered for another reason: pain during intercourse. This is not a direct cause of infertility, but it hinders conception by restricting intercourse. During coitus the man's penis, especially if it is large, will press against the cervix and gently push the uterus up a short way inside the pelvis. If that natural movement is restricted by retroversion, some deep discomfort may result. Occasionally this can be relieved by the woman being on top during intercourse, allowing the uterus to fall fowards under the effects of gravity. That, at least, is the theory.

Where a retroverted uterus causes discomfort a device (plastic or rubber pessary) can be placed in the vagina to tilt the womb forward. If that brings relief, the gynaecologist might then offer an operation to shorten the round ligaments and permanently antevert the retroverted uterus. (Another possibility that will cross the doctor's mind when a woman who previously experienced pain-free sex complains of deep pain during intercourse is endometriosis, which we discussed on pp. 74–6.) When pregnancy occurs in a retroverted uterus, the uterus expands naturally inside the pelvis and then pushes outside the pelvis in the normal way. In the past women with retroversion were asked to rest lying face down to encourage the womb forwards during early pregnancy; there is little evidence that this is of much value, but it might give the woman a good excuse to rest while her partner gets on with the household chores!

10

Reversal of sterilization

An increasingly common cause of infertility for which both men and women are seeking medical help is sterilization. To many, especially to those who long for a child but have never been able to produce one, it may seem incongruous that people who have been sterilized, usually after they have had two or more children, should suddenly change their minds and want more. Obviously, the object of sterilizing a man or a woman is to terminate his or her fertility, effectively and permanently, and nobody should be sterilized unless they are absolutely sure they do not want more children. There is no guarantee that a sterilization operation can be successfully reversed, and any doctor who agrees to sterilize someone will first make certain that the patient understands this; if after discussion (usually with both partners in the relationship) there is any doubt in either the man's or the woman's mind, it is best to defer the operation.

Why it may be necessary

Nevertheless, it is perhaps inevitable that a small number of people who have been sterilized come forward to request a reversal procedure. This often arises from a change in family circumstances: people who had considered their families complete may be widowed or divorced and then remarry, wanting to have children from the new relationship. Or it might be that a child has been lost through accident or illness—a natural reaction to the tragedy of a child's death is the desire to have another.

Thorough pre-operative counselling does ensure that the percentage of people wanting a reversal remains low, but the increasing popularity of sterilization leaves in its wake a small but steady stream of men and women hoping for a chance of remedying their now involuntary infertility. Sterilization can—sometimes—be reversed, and in this chapter we shall look at what this involves. The implications are, incidentally, of relevance to general infertility work. When performing a reversal operation the surgeon faces largely the same problems as when operating to repair blocked or damaged Fallopian tubes or blocked or damaged tubes inside the testis; different techniques are being experimented with, and the experience gained from the one operation is of value to the other.

Sterilization of women Three main types of sterilization procedure are used for women; of these, some are much easier to reverse than others. It is important to remember that all these techniques are designed for maximum efficiency of sterilization and not their potential for reversal. Recently, however, and in the face of the steady number of women requesting reversal, doctors have tended to choose those techniques which are effective methods of sterilization, yet do offer a reasonable chance of reversal.

The most common method of sterilization is still an open operation, in which a small incision is made into the abdominal wall to reveal the Fallopian tubes, which are then cut. As the cut ends of the tubes would frequently recanalize (join up again) if simply left hanging close to one another, a variety of techniques is used to keep the ends apart. The tubes may simply be tied off with absorbable sutures, or more complex procedures may be employed; for example, the cut ends may be buried in adjacent structures such as the broad ligament (the fold of tissue enveloping the tubes and the uterus).

The second most common method of sterilization is diathermy (electrical cautery) of the tubes, using the laparoscope for direct vision and a separate pair of forceps connected to an electrical current. The heat produced by the current causes the tubes to coagulate, and much of their length is destroyed.

The third form of sterilization is becoming increasingly popular and will probably supersede the first and second methods almost completely in the course of time. It

Methods of female sterilization

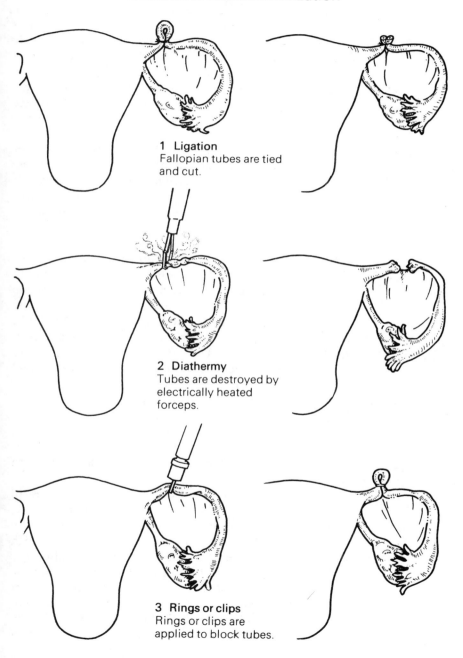

1 Ligation
Fallopian tubes are tied and cut.

2 Diathermy
Tubes are destroyed by electrically heated forceps.

3 Rings or clips
Rings or clips are applied to block tubes.

consists of blocking off each tube with clips or rings, again using a laparoscope for direct vision and a special 'gun' to apply the clips or rings.

A fourth method of sterilization, but one which is much less commonly used, is internal blockage of the tubes; this may be performed by means of an intrauterine implant to block the 'horns' of the uterus (cornual occlusion) or by sealing the entrance of the tubes to the uterus under direct vision using a hysteroscope passed through the vagina.

Chances of successful reversal

The chances of reversing a female sterilization operation depend on the amount of damage to the Fallopian tubes. Quite obviously, if a large portion of the tubes is damaged, as may occur in the diathermy technique, then the chances of reversal are correspondingly small. Similarly, in another method of sterilization known as fimbriectomy (rarely used today), where the fimbriae or finger-like fronds of the tubes near the ovary are removed altogether, there is little hope of returning fertility. Doctors are now moving away from the destructive diathermy technique towards the application of small clips or rings. The technique has not been in use as long as the other methods, and at present relatively few reversal attempts have been made, but the results of these are very encouraging (many centres are now reporting success rates of between 50 and 95 per cent, depending on the location of the repair). The majority of sterilization reversals performed so far have been on women whose Fallopian tubes have been cut and their ends buried and the experts regularly performing reversal operations can now achieve at least a 50 per cent success rate in those women who have a reasonable length of tube remaining.

A variety of factors affect the chances of successful reversal, both anatomical and physiological. For example, a tube which is not only divided but seriously affected by infection is unlikely to function again. The point at which the tube has been cut, blocked, or destroyed is also very significant. The normal Fallopian tube begins within the wall of the uterus and then emerges as a rather narrow part of the tube called the isthmus. The isthmus soon widens out into the ampullary (bulb-like) part of the tube. As you can imagine, a sterilization performed at the junction of

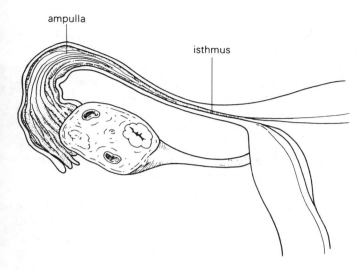

ampulla

isthmus

Diameters of the Fallopian tube at the isthmus and the ampulla are markedly different. If sterilization is carried out by clips or rings applied to the isthmus, subsequent reversal has more chance of success.

the isthmus and ampulla will give two ends of tube with quite different diameters, and re-joining them poses a difficult surgical problem. Experimental work with animals (mostly rabbits), particularly that performed at the University of Texas, San Antonio, and at the Hammersmith Hospital, London, shows that it is technically easiest to rejoin the tubes at the isthmus region, i.e., close to the uterus. This conclusion is supported by clinical experience. As the calibre of the isthmic portion is more or less uniform, the internal diameter of the two segments of tube will normally be similar. Knowing this, the doctor aims to apply a sterilizing clip or to divide the tubes about 1–2cm (½–1in) from the uterus.

The technical problems of reversal operations and ways to overcome them are still subjects for debate among surgeons. Many feel that the operations can be performed with the naked eye using fine nylon suture materials to stitch the two tube ends together. Another group of surgeons favours the use of operating microscopes, with time-consuming microsurgical dissections. Although in theory it would seem that the use of microsurgical techniques would be the most logical approach, the advantages of such techniques are at present not overwhelming. One significant fact, however, is that fewer ectopic

Technical considerations

pregnancies have been recorded following tubal surgery using micro-techniques, and although the pregnancy rate following salpingostomy operations (opening up a blocked Fallopian tube at the end nearest the ovary) is no different after microsurgical techniques, there is an improvement in the results of sterilization reversals.

Our present knowledge of the normal physiology and functioning of the Fallopian tube, with its complex system of egg transport, is still limited, and the surgeon can aim only to join together the delicate sections of tube as best he can, ensuring that there is an adequate blood supply and a relatively infection-free environment in which healing can take place. Many surgeons who were disappointed when post-operative fibrosis (scar-tissue formation) and adhesions hindered successful reversal decided to give their patients anti-inflammatory steroid injections or tablets after the operation, but experimental evidence now shows that steroids are unlikely to prevent such complications. In an effort to maintain the tiny canal within the Fallopian tube, surgeons frequently proceeded by placing a very thin nylon splint (similar to fishing line) down the tube and joining the tube over the splint, pulling the tubes together over the nylon like the sleeves of a coat. It is now thought that although such splints represent a great help in surgical technique, they may damage the delicate lining of the tube and many surgeons do not now leave them in for a few days after the operation.

A great concern of gynaecologists in performing these operations to re-join the Fallopian tubes, as in normal Fallopian tube surgery, is to reduce the possibility of an ectopic pregnancy. This occurs when a fertilized ovum fails to descend into the womb, but instead embeds itself in the Fallopian tube, where it begins to grow and develop. An ectopic pregnancy usually causes copious bleeding and endangers the woman's life. It is postulated that the scar existing where the two ends of tube are joined may encourage a fertilized ovum to implant there. In order to minimize this chance surgeons take care to remove any fibrous tissue at the ends of the tubes so that they join only fresh and healthy tissue, which reduces the risk of any further scar tissue forming at the junction. Fortunately, however, the occurrence of ectopic pregnancy after a reversal operation has become uncommon, although it was as high as 20 per cent before the widespread use of microsurgical techniques employing fine suture materials.

It is very interesting to note that tests performed on women who have been unable to conceive after a reversal operation show that the majority of them do in fact have open tubes. Although the operations must therefore be considered surgical successes, they are functional failures since the women are unable to conceive. The reason for this may be that the operations damage the tube lining. While a great deal remains to be discovered about how the Fallopian tubes function, we do know that where the lining of the tube contains a reduced number of cells bearing tiny hairs known as cilia, normal transportation of the ovum is impaired. At the Hammersmith Hospital in London small samples (biopsies) of the tube lining have been examined under a scanning electron microscope to assess the number of these cilia-bearing cells with a view to predicting the chances of pregnancy after tubal surgery, whether performed to reverse sterilization or for other reasons. This remains an experimental research procedure for the moment.

Technical versus functional success

However, the results of the reversal operations are improving year by year and we can hope with some degree of confidence that the more thoughtful and less aggressive approach to sterilization will in the future enhance even further the chances of reversal without sacrificing the effectiveness of the sterilization.

Incidentally, there have been a very few attempts at Fallopian-tube transplantation—using the tubes of either an animal or another woman to replace those of a woman who has completely lost her own tubal function. One such transplant took place in Melbourne, Australia, and despite great efforts to avoid the problem of tissue rejection which occur in any transplant—through the use of immunosuppressive drugs and exceptionally close tissue-typing, the transplant being from one sister to another—the operation was not a success, and a subsequent pregnancy was not achieved. The team involved has been discouraged from repeating the experiment.

Active research continues to look for new ways of

providing a completely reversible method of sterilization, and new methods such as placing the fimbriae in a silastic cap, like a little hood, are currently under investigation. It is possible that if in vitro fertilization systems become more available and more effective, there may be no need to perform reversal of sterilization operations. However, at the present time IVF may offer some hope for those women for whom reversal is not possible.

Reversal of male sterilization

In the United Kingdom several studies have shown that between 2 per cent and 3 per cent of vasectomized men request reversals. In the United States a survey in 1980 estimated the proportion to be 6.7 per cent. In both countries the numbers of men requesting reversal operations are increasing. In a study of men who had requested reversal of vasectomy, carried out at Charing Cross Hospital in London and reported in 1982, it was found that a greater number of requests came from men who had been under 35 years of age at the time of vasectomy and who were more likely to have been divorced, especially if there had been a teenage pregnancy. Almost all the men in the survey who had requested reversal emphasized that vasectomy had been carried out at a time of crisis, when they were convinced that sterilization was the only way out of their difficulties. Many men thought that the operation had been carried out too quickly. Some had had the operation within one week of their first enquiry, one within 24 hours of a telephone call.

The operation of vasectomy simply consists of dividing each vas deferens—the tubes which conduct the sperm from the testes up past the seminal vesicles, through the prostate gland and out through the penis via the urethra (see p. 52). The operation is normally performed under local anaesthetic through a very small incision in the upper part of the scrotum. The ends of the tubes are usually bent back on themselves and tied down.

As a means of sterilization, vasectomy has a very high success rate. When it comes to reversal however there is, as in the case of women, a disparity between the rates of technical and functional success. Technical success is achieved by the restoration of normal sperm counts at seminalysis after the tubes have been rejoined, whereas

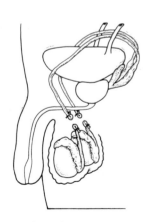

Male sterilization (vasectomy) involves simple tying back of the vasa deferentia.

functional success is defined by occurrence of a pregnancy afterwards. There have been various claims of technical success ranging from 38 to 90 per cent, but the respective rates of functional success vary between 19 and 59 per cent. Many theories have been advanced to account for this disparity, including immunological and hormonal factors, but as with the Fallopian tubes in women, we do not yet know enough about the physiology of these tubes and associated organs completely to explain these failures.

All scar tissue is removed and the two cut ends of the vasa deferentia are brought together over a thin nylon splint, which is usually removed some days after the operation. As with female reversals, surgeons have varying views about the use of splints, the type of sutures used and post-operative management; most however seem to place a great deal of emphasis on adequate bed-rest following the operation. It is known that the passage of spermatozoa through the newly joined tube does not help the chances of success, and some doctors use drugs before the operation to suppress the formation of sperm, while some remove sperm at the time of operation from the epididymis, where they are stored on top of the testes. Once again, although microsurgical techniques are favoured, some good results are obtained simply by using the naked eye.

The reversal procedure

Following reversal of male sterilization initial sperm counts are usually low in density (5–10 million per ml) with some impairment of motility. Subsequent specimens usually show progressive improvement in sperm density, viability and motility. In many cases sperm density remains low and this is frequently seen in patients who have been sterilized for some considerable time, such as ten or more years; after such a long period of inactivity, the rate of sperm production is understandably decreased.

On the whole, the rate of functional success after reversal of vasectomy is encouraging and suggests that a sterilized man has a reasonable chance of return to fertility. However, there is no reason at the moment for altering the basis of vasectomy counselling, in which applicants are asked to accept it may not be possible to reverse the operation and are asked to consider it as irreversible.

11

In vitro fertilization

In 1978 Patrick Steptoe, a gynaecologist working with Robert Edwards, a scientist, successfully delivered Louise Brown—the world's first baby produced as an ovum fertilized outside of her mother's body. Since this remarkable achievement there has been considerable development of this technique and treatment facilities have been established in various parts of the United Kingdom. Considerable expertise has also been developed in Australia and the United States of America.

The basic technique is simple to understand. Several ripe ova (eggs) are removed from the woman's ovaries and then mixed with especially prepared spermatozoa (see p. 139). The spermatozoa fertilize the ova and several embryos develop. These are then checked by an expert embryologist and several of them are inserted into the woman's uterus. Any unused embryos can be frozen and stored for later use. Fingers are then crossed in the hope that one or more of the embryos will implant into the lining of the uterus and a successful pregnancy will ensue.

What is IVF?

Various scientific terms have been applied to this process including 'extracorporeal fertilization', i.e., fertilization outside of the body (the Latin word *corpus*, the body, being the derivation of corporeal); and the now often used term 'in vitro fertilization' i.e., fertilization in a test-tube or glass dish, from the Latin word *vitrum*, which means glass. The opposite of 'in vitro' is 'in vivo', meaning in the living body. In vitro fertilization has become the most popular term with the medical profession and the method is frequently referred to as 'IVF'. The popular term 'test-tube baby' is misleading, since only the fertilization of the ovum and its development during the first day or two takes place in a dish in the laboratory; thereafter the developing embryo is placed in its mother's body and the baby produced completes his or her growth in the normal way.

The world's first test-tube baby was born by Caesarean section because of pregnancy complications unrelated to conception by in vitro fertilization. Women who become pregnant by this method are subsequently cared for by obstetricians like any other pregnant woman and do not have to be delivered by Caesarean section just because they are carrying an IVF produced pregnancy. The majority will deliver vaginally in the normal way. Having said that, as you would expect and would wish, any obstetrician looking after a woman who has had extensive tests and treatment for infertility and has finally become pregnant by IVF is likely to be very careful and extra cautious in managing the pregnancy, labour and delivery.

Suitability for IVF

The majority of couples who are being referred for IVF are those where the only major problem is the woman's Fallopian tubes. Most of these will have been blocked or rendered ineffective by previous infection or surgery, and often tubal surgery will have been performed earlier in an attempt to unblock the tubes and been unsuccessful. A woman who has had both her tubes removed after ectopic pregnancies would also find that IVF is her only chance of becoming pregnant.

Another group of couples being referred for IVF is those with 'unexplained infertility'. These couples will have been extensively investigated in the past and no major cause for their lack of success found. Many doctors now feel that couples with unexplained infertility who have been trying to conceive for over five years should be recommended for IVF. It is possible that defects in the cervical mucus and/or the transport of spermatozoa up to the ova in the Fallopian tubes is the cause of some unexplained infertility. Studies in Australia and Britain suggest that successful IVF is possible in unexplained infertility and the chance of pregnancy quite high. Several of my patients with unexplained infertility have conceived whilst waiting to be considered for IVF and it is interesting to speculate if being on the waiting list for IVF confers a beneficial effect itself! Probably not when the statistics are analysed but in every case where it has happened there has been great jubilation.

IVF and male infertility When Mr Steptoe announced the technique was possible there was considerable hope that men with very low sperm counts (oligospermia) might be able to be helped by IVF. It was hoped that just a few viable spermatozoa would be needed to fertilize the normal ova in the laboratory by the IVF method. Unfortunately, although there have been some successes with selected cases, IVF using the partner's sperm in these cases has not yet fulfilled all our hopes. It is likely that in addition to the reduced numbers of sperm produced by these men, the sperm may not be of sufficient quality to effect successful fertilization, but in these cases donor sperm can be used instead. Thus a woman whose Fallopian tubes are damaged or absent and whose partner is oligospermic would find artificial insemination unsuccessful, but may be helped by IVF using donor sperm. We all hope that further research into male infertility may bring more encouraging results in its treatment by IVF.

The need for in vitro fertilization Dr Michael Hull and his colleagues in the University of Bristol recently estimated the need for in vitro fertilization in the general population, as he reported in the *British Medical Journal*. Among his patients unexplained infertility gave rise to the largest group (28 per cent) of couples who may need IVF. Nearly 20 per cent of women with tubal damage had become pregnant by other means, leaving approximately 80 per cent suitable for in vitro fertilization. He thought that about a quarter of those patients with unexplained infertility had prolonged infertility, in excess of five years, and would be suitable for IVF. Adding the two groups together, about 18 per cent of all infertile couples may be suitable for IVF and this, he calculated, would mean about 216 couples undergoing IVF each year per million of the total population. He mentioned, of course, that not all couples would want to go for IVF but to compensate for this, some couples would want a second or subsequent child by IVF later on.

Usually couples selected for IVF will have come to the end of extensive investigations and treatments in a hospital-based infertility clinic. The implications of the technique are fully discussed with the couple and many questions posed and answered.

Referral to an IVF centre

The doctor in the infertility clinic will then write a long letter of application for IVF to the nearest centre offering the technique. The letter would summarize all the medical history of the couple, including clinical findings, investigation results and treatments already tried. If all the selection criteria of the particular IVF centre are satisfied then the couple are placed on the waiting list. There may well be supplementary questions asked of the referring specialist by the IVF centre to clear up any outstanding points, such as missing reports, suggested other treatments to be tried first, etc. Selection criteria for some IVF centres include an upper age limit, as the chance of success with IVF is poor when the age of the woman exceeds 38 to 40 years, and some centres only offer treatment to couples living in the vicinity. When the accepted couples approach the top of the waiting list they will be invited to the IVF centre to discuss treatment. It should be recognized, however, that the waiting time could be as long as three years for National Health Service centres.

Remember that gynaecologists offering IVF treatment are not purely technicians who carry out IVF with no questions asked. They are infertility experts themselves and will wish to ensure that all orthodox investigations and treatments have been completed before resorting to IVF. They may thus recommend further tests and/or treatments themselves before offering IVF. Only when they are satisfied that IVF is appropriate will they make arrangements for it to be carried out.

If a woman has ovaries which are buried in adhesions following severe pelvic infections or post-operative scarring, she may undergo surgery to clear the surfaces of the ovaries. This could have been done already at the time of previous tubal surgery, but if there is any doubt that

Preparing the pelvis for IVF

adhesions may have occurred again a preparatory operation may be required. In the majority of women a laparoscopy at least will have been performed before referral for IVF takes place, so the state of the pelvis will be known.

Preparing the ovaries

One of the improvements in technique which has led to great success in IVF is the placing of more than one fertilized ovum (embryo) into the uterus. Without stimulation only one ovum could be removed during each cycle, so it has become necessary to stimulate the ripening of several follicles so that up to half a dozen ova can be collected at the same time. (See p. 109 for a detailed explanation of follicle stimulation.)

The details may vary from one IVF unit to another but a common system would involve giving 150 mgs of clomiphene daily from days 2 to 6 of the menstrual cycle and then human menopausal gonadotrophin (FSH) injections, say two ampoules daily from days 5 to 9 of the cycle. This will cause several follicles to swell and these can be measured and monitored by ultrasound scanning of the ovaries. When the leading follicle has reached a good size (e.g. 18mm), an injection of human chorionic gonadotrophin (HCG), which mimics luteinizing hormone, is given for final ripening.

'Ovum harvest'

There are two current ways of performing ovum harvest (in other words, collecting the ova)—one using laparoscopy and the other using ultrasound location.

The technique introduced by Mr Steptoe involved performing a laparoscopy in order to view the stimulated ovaries and, using a fine, narrow bore needle introduced through the abdominal wall connected to a reservoir containing suitable medium fluid, the ova could be sucked out of their follicles under direct vision through the laparoscope. The laparoscopy is performed under general anaesthesia (fully asleep), as usual, which adds considerably to the disturbance of the woman and the cost of the overall procedure. There is a small surgical and anaesthetic risk too. The physical and emotional stresses induced by the procedure may be traumatic enough to prejudice the chances of successful implantation of the embryos.

The technique of in vitro fertilization

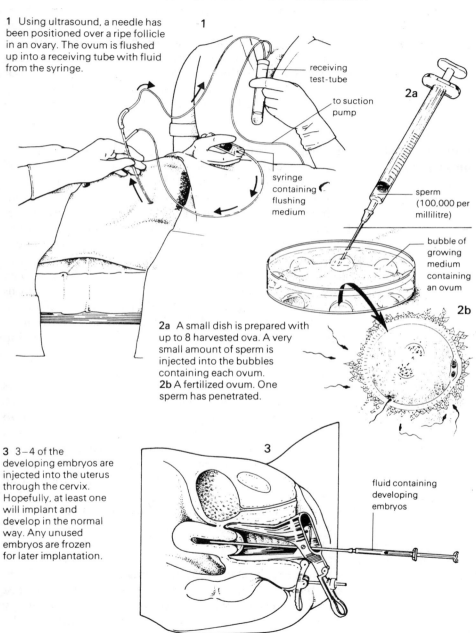

1 Using ultrasound, a needle has been positioned over a ripe follicle in an ovary. The ovum is flushed up into a receiving tube with fluid from the syringe.

receiving test-tube

to suction pump

syringe containing flushing medium

sperm (100,000 per millilitre)

bubble of growing medium containing an ovum

2a A small dish is prepared with up to 8 harvested ova. A very small amount of sperm is injected into the bubbles containing each ovum.
2b A fertilized ovum. One sperm has penetrated.

3 3–4 of the developing embryos are injected into the uterus through the cervix. Hopefully, at least one will implant and develop in the normal way. Any unused embryos are frozen for later implantation.

fluid containing developing embryos

The other method of ovum harvest involves ultrasound scanning of the pelvis and location of each follicle. A thin bore needle can then be introduced through the abdominal wall, traversing the bladder and into the ovarian follicles. Using ultrasound guidance the ova can be sucked out of their follicles. General anaesthesia is not usually necessary for this; it can be performed using local anaesthesia, which numbs the skin of the abdomen where the needle is inserted.

Fertilization and implantation

Having successfully removed the ova they are then mixed with especially prepared spermatozoa provided by the partner (or by a donor in special cases). Preparation of the spermatozoa is necessary to mimic the 'capacitation' which takes place in the cervical mucus as the sperm travel through up to the Fallopian tubes. Certain proteins need to be washed from the surface of the spermatozoa before they are able to penetrate the cell wall of the ovum in order to fuse with the nucleus and effect fertilization. The raw spermatozoa are therefore washed in special solutions to remove these proteins. These capacitated spermatozoa are then mixed with the collected ova and fertilization allowed to take place. As the resulting embryos develop they are checked carefully to ensure they are dividing properly.

Approximately 40 hours after fertilization the embryos will have divided twice and be at the four-cell stage (see p. 19), ready for implantation into the uterus. Usually two or three or more embryos are used and any embryos which are not used could be stored for later reimplantation, if the first attempt is unsuccessful. The developing embryos are injected through the cervix into the uterine cavity.

There then follows an anxious time until the next period is due. Pregnancy—that is successful implantation of at least one embryo into the lining of the womb—can be checked using a blood test which measures the very early rise in human chorionic gonadotrophin (HCG) in the bloodstream. The more traditional pregnancy test measures the level of HCG in the urine but will not usually be positive until several weeks after implantation—the blood test gives a much earlier result.

For couples with unexplained infertility who have re- **Fertilization within the**
ligious or other reasons for declining fertilization outside **Fallopian tube**
the body, as in current IVF systems, a new technique has
been developed in Australia which may be of help. In this
method laparoscopy is performed and a fine tube is
introduced into the fimbrial end of the Fallopian tube.
This allows a small quantity of capacitated spermatozoa to
be injected into the Fallopian tube; this is followed by an
air bubble. A harvested ovum is then injected alongside
the air bubble. Fertilization takes place in the Fallopian
tube as usual and the embryo later moves down into the
cavity of the uterus in the usual way. Pregnancy rates have
been satisfactory and the theoretical risk of producing an
excessive number of ectopic pregnancies (with implantation occurring in the Fallopian tube and not in the uterus)
does not appear in practice. This technique may be of use
in couples with 'unexplained infertility'—unfortunately it
does require the use of laparoscopy. The technique is
frequently referred to as G.I.F.T., which stands for
Gamete Intra-Fallopian Transfer, although the term
T.S.E.T., Tubal Sperm–Egg Transfer, is gaining
currency.

It is difficult to predict the chance of success of IVF in each **Chances of success**
individual case, but most IVF units keep a close check on **with IVF**
their overall pregnancy rates. Since the birth of Louise
Brown in 1978 there has been a steady improvement in
success rates, one of the major strides forward being the
use of more than one embryo for implantation—despite
the much increased chance of multiple pregnancy. One of
the major problems yet to be solved is the high miscarriage
rate following successful implantation.

In order to give some idea of current practice the
following figures are frequently quoted. Approximately
25–30 per cent of IVF attempts result in a pregnancy, i.e.,
successful implantation, but only 10–15 per cent will end
with a viable baby.

Comparisons are often made between the similar
overall results of tubal surgery and those of IVF. These are
frequently not valid. Some patients may be totally
unsuitable for tubal surgery, IVF being their only chance,
such as after removal of both Fallopian tubes. On the other

hand, other patients for whom IVF may be suitable as well as tubal surgery may find that tubal surgery facilities are more accessible than those of IVF. Preferably the pros and cons of each technique should be considered in each individual case with an infertility specialist and the right treatment chosen.

Availability of IVF facilities

At the present time the majority of what few IVF centres there are in the United Kingdom are provided by university academic departments of gynaecology. These may work in conjunction with the National Health Service or with medical facilities provided by private organizations such as American private hospital groups. The National Health Service has provided very little support so far and there are no major plans to introduce widespread NHS IVF treatment centres.

IVF treatment is very labour intensive—it is a seven days per week, 24 hours per day service. Laboratory standards and facilities need to be of the highest standards and attract appropriate costs. Some of the academic units ask NHS patients for a nominal contribution such as £100; the academic units usually take private patients too at full cost. Costs of private IVF treatment vary between £1,000 and £2,000 for each attempt. Those using ultrasound–guided, rather than laparoscopic, ovum harvest may well be found towards the less expensive end of the price range. The demand for IVF has been so great that units have been compelled to restrict patients by age and proximity to the centre. Waiting lists for private patients are usually only a month or two—waiting lists for other patients are often between one and two years. With many units refusing to take women over 37 or 38 years of age it is sensible to refer early for IVF rather than later if orthodox infertility treatment has failed.

Centres currently involved with IVF treatment are located in Edinburgh, Dundee, Manchester, Nottingham, Sheffield, Birmingham; Mr Patrick Steptoe has established his treatment centre just outside Cambridge at Bourne Hall. In London IVF centres are located at the Royal Free Hospital in Hampstead, King's College Hospital in Camberwell, St Bartholomew's Hospital in the City, Hammersmith Hospital in West London, and

Chelsea Hospital for Women. Within the private sector Mr Ian Craft provides facilities at the Wellington Hospital in St John's Wood and Dr Bridgett Mason at the Hallam Medical Centre in Central London. (She also works in association with King's College Hospital.)

The future of IVF

Several other hospitals in London and other parts of the country are considering plans to establish IVF facilities. Interest within the private sector has been shown in setting up new centres in both existing private hospitals and in new purpose-built premises. Several established IVF centres have taken on extra staff to improve treatment facilities. Against this is the gloomy news that some centres are so overwhelmed with requests that they are trying to close their waiting lists completely, such is the number of couples who now want IVF treatment. It is highly unlikely that IVF facilities will ever meet the demand in the foreseeable future.

The ethical questions

IVF treatment has raised several ethical questions but not as many as those surrounding the possibility of performing badly-needed research on human embryos. Doctors involved with IVF are members of the Voluntary Licensing Authority chaired by Dame Mary Donaldson, former Lord Mayor of London and nurse at the Middlesex Hospital. This provides an internal control of ethical standards. A committee under the leadership of Dame Mary Warnock has made recommendations to set up guidelines and controls on both IVF treatment and the regulation of embryo research. Within the House of Commons private members bills have been debated which have been intended to introduce statutory controls over IVF treatment and embryo research. Opinion is currently divided between those who feel that research into causes of congenital diseases such as cystic fibrosis is justified on embryos up to 14 days old and those who feel that research on embryos is immoral. It is hoped that facilities for IVF treatment will not be caught in the crossfire.

12

Artificial insemination

Artificial insemination is most often associated with the veterinary world, where it has been standard practice for many years; however, a gradual change in attitude has led to greater interest in using this technique to treat certain cases of subfertility by artificially inseminating the wife with her husband's semen (AIH) or that of a donor (AID). Until relatively recently there was little documentation of these techniques—the extent to which they had been performed, the results and the problems which went with them—as this had been left to individual practitioners with an interest in the subject. Over the past decade a considerable amount of facts and figures has been collected and in this chapter I hope to give you a balanced appraisal of the current knowledge of the procedure.

The history of artificial insemination We can go right back to the year 220 AD when the Talmud questioned the paternity of a child born to a woman who, it was alleged, was accidentally fertilized in bath water! Whether this was an ingenious 'cover-up' story on behalf of an adulterous woman we do not know, but debate about the paternity issue still continues over 1700 years later in a modified form—more of this further on. One of the first recorded instances of artificial insemination performed on livestock came in the fourteenth century when the ingenious Sheik Hegira inseminated his mares with semen, obtained clandestinely from the prize stallion of a rival. But the first recorded pregnancy and delivery of a child conceived by AIH was made in 1790 by John Hunter, the great anatomist and surgeon of St George's Hospital, London (my old medical school). This was followed in the United States by Marion Sims in 1866. In the same year, Montegazzi introduced the idea of a 'sperm bank'. In 1890 Robert Dickinson began using AID (using donor semen), although his work was carried out in secret.

The demand for artificial insemination, and especially for AID, is increasing today as a result of the generally disappointing success rate in the treatment of male infertility, combined with a marked decrease in the availability of babies for adoption. Estimates of the proportion of marriages which have subfertility problems range from 9 to 15 per cent, and various studies have concluded that the cause rests with the male partner alone in between 10 and 50 per cent of these cases. A British study suggests that in the UK 16,000 marriages will be infertile each year because of infertility in the husband alone. It is estimated that in the United States 6–10,000 babies are now born by AID each year; in Britain the figure is about 6,000 babies per year, and in both countries the numbers are rising steadily.

Current demand

One of the situations in which AIH is recommended is where the husband has oligospermia (produces a low level of spermatozoa); unfortunately, the results have not produced a vast improvement in the pregnancy rate, though successes have been achieved, and it is often worth a try. Perhaps in the future more hope will be offered by in vitro fertilization in these cases, as mentioned in the previous chapter. AIH is, however, of particular value in situations where the sperm count is normal but where normal intercourse is difficult, for example, through impotence, paraplegia, etc. Frozen semen stored in banks (cryopreservation) may allow later parenthood to men undergoing removal of the testicles (orchidectomy) or radiotherapy to the testes, for instance, in cases of cancer of the testicles.

Artificial insemination by husband (AIH)

AID is chosen primarily when the husband is completely infertile. However, the procedure is sometimes requested to avoid passing on some inherited disease such as Rhesus

Reasons for using AID

factor incompatibility, cystic fibrosis, diabetes, haemo-philia, Huntington's disease, muscular dystrophy, and other genetically transmissible diseases. In one survey in the United States at least 10 per cent of the participating doctors had provided AID for single women in order to 'provide natural children to women without a male partner'. However, this is still fairly uncommon on both sides of the Atlantic.

Selection of donors

The selection of sperm donors is a particular problem and the procedure varies considerably. In Britain the Royal College of Obstetricians and Gynaecologists recently produced a Study Group proposal suggesting that before semen is collected a potential donor should be interviewed and a full medical and family history obtained, a general physical examination performed, and that he should then be asked to sign a form to state that he is fully aware of how the semen will be used. Most practitioners recommend extra medical tests on donors to exclude diabetes, chromosome abnormalities, Rhesus factor problems and syphilis. Donors are now being screened for infection with the AIDS virus, as well. Similar guidelines are followed in the United States and according to one large study 62 per cent of doctors used medical students or hospital residents as donors, 10 per cent used other university or graduate students, and 18 per cent used both. 10 per cent selected donors from military academies, husbands of obstetric patients, hospital personnel, and friends of the physician. Some doctors try to match donors to recipient parents in terms of stature, hair and eye coloration, etc. It is not usual for any one doctor to be used for more than five or six pregnancies as doctors are aware of the undesirable possibility of subsequent marriages between offspring of the same donor. Incidentally, donors are usually paid a nominal sum, £5 to £10 per ejaculate is not uncommon. In Britain there are several commercial sperm banks and a few operated by academic departments of medical schools, but none run purely by the NHS.

The Pregnancy Advisory Service, a registered charity, offers artificial insemination facilities. They claim that AID has been practised in the United Kingdom for fifty years and that currently at least 2,500 babies a year are conceived in this way. PAS understands that their fees are the lowest in the private sector, charging £60 for counselling and examination and £35 for two inseminations per month.

How it is done

For both AID and AIH, the semen is collected (usually by masturbation) in a polythene vial, and a small drop is taken for analysis. Fresh semen is marginally more likely to produce a pregnancy than a cryopreserved specimen, but for convenience in most centres the semen is frozen for later use. A preserving mixture, which may contain glycerol, egg yolk, fructose, and citrate in distilled water is added to the semen. It is then cooled gently in the vapour of liquid nitrogen and stored immersed in that liquid at a temperature of around −196°C.

Insemination takes place on the day before ovulation is expected. In a woman with fairly regular cycles, this can be deduced from temperature and menstrual charts. If ovulation cannot be predicted with any certainty multiple inseminations may be made say every two or three days at the midcycle time. If this is not thought to be reliable enough in a particular case, ovulation can be measured more accurately by hormone levels in the urine each day. Just before ovulation a surge of luteinizing hormone and a rise in the level of oestrogens occur (see p. 18). Some doctors use fertility drugs to stimulate ovulation if pregnancy has not occurred after a few attempts (see p. 107).

At insemination the woman lies on her side or on her back with her legs in stirrups and her buttocks raised up to encourage the semen to collect near to the cervix. The cervix is exposed with a bivalved speculum (as is used in taking a cervical smear). Although techniques of insemination vary slightly, the usual procedure is to place about 1 ml of semen into the mucus in the cervical canal with a plastic tube and syringe. The woman usually rests in that position for about half an hour. Some doctors also spray a little semen on to the surface of the cervix and upper end of the vagina, or fit a plastic cap over the cervix to retain the semen and allow the woman to rise immediately. The cap is removed after eight hours by the woman herself.

Pregnancy rates following artificial insemination do not

seem to vary a great deal from centre to centre, which is perhaps surprising. In Britain most centres report a 20 per cent pregnancy rate for AIH (although it rises to 85 per cent in cases where the husband's seminalysis is good and it is performed because of difficulties with intercourse). The average success rates for AID are between 55 per cent and 78 per cent (66 per cent if fresh semen is used and 41 per cent if frozen). Approximately 85–90 per cent of women usually conceive within six months of insemination—about 20 per cent in the first menstrual cycle, and 50–70 per cent by the third. The 10–15 per cent of women who do not conceive after repeated inseminations may well require investigation. It is pleasing to note that, almost certainly as a result of preselection of donors and the elimination of many potential problems, miscarriage, ectopic pregnancy and congenital abnormalities occur less frequently in pregnancies produced by AID than in normal pregnancies.

Psychological factors It is not difficult to imagine that the psychological effects of artificial insemination on both husband and wife can be very considerable. Studies carried out in the United States in the early 1960s show that psychological disturbance is not uncommon both before and after the procedure. The psychological stresses must be particularly great in the case of AID. Many a man would resent the idea that his wife should carry another man's baby, even though the donor remains completely unknown to both husband and wife. On the other hand, he might not object to the idea, or might overcome his reservations in recognition of the fact that AID represents the only chance that his wife will have to bear a much-wanted baby.

Doctors are well aware of the potential stresses these factors may cause, and will not offer to perform artificial insemination until the couple have had some sort of counselling. More recent studies have shown that where careful counselling has taken place, the risk of psychological disturbance or strain is greatly reduced. Most doctors make a judgement during an initial interview with the couple, based on their attitudes, about the need for counselling. Specialist counselling is sometimes available, but it is by no means routine.

The decision to have AID is obviously a difficult one for both partners. Husbands tend to feel guilty, distressed by being unable to 'prove their manhood' or to fulfil the expectations of family and society, or feel that they cannot become 'a real father' to an AID child. Women also experience a conflict between sharing the man's failure and their own pride. However, experience shows that most couples who request AID sort these problems out; they express a positive interest in the procedure, considering that it allows the woman to experience pregnancy and that the child will inherit characteristics of the mother at least. The increasing difficulty of adopting newborn infants may well influence a couple to choose AID.

Is an AID child legitimate?

In Britain, and especially in England, there is very little statute or case law concerning the legal standing of children produced by AID. It has been deemed by some that the child is illegitimate, because a legitimate child is defined as the product of a married couple. AID itself is not illegal. A Ciba Foundation Study in the early 1970s made several proposals concerning the legal implications of AID, including one that the doctor should maintain a record of the donor's identity. This raises the difficult problem of donor anonymity. Further suggestions were that the description of the male parent at the registration of the birth of an AID child should be amended, and that the husband and wife should make a joint application to adopt the child. In 1973 the Peel Committee recommended that a child born as a result of donor insemination should be regarded as legitimate provided that the mother and husband had both consented to AID beforehand, and that at registration of the birth the husband should be deemed to be the father.

At the time of writing the legal position in most parts of the world remains confused and I can only pass on the conclusion of the Ciba Foundation Study mentioned above: that there is a definite demand for AID and the technique is here to stay—at least until there is a vast improvement in the outlook for the treatment of infertile men—and the law should regulate the subject in a way which is acceptable to society, rather than inhibit, or even prohibit, the continued use of this technique.

13

What now?

In this concluding section I would like to consider the situation facing couples for whom the chances of having a baby, conceived of both parents, are either nil or remote, after all the necessary tests have been performed and all the relevant treatments available have been tried. One possibility that many such couples might consider is adoption; another is to resign themselves to childlessness, or 'child-free living' as it has been called.

The end of the road

The more experienced a doctor is the less likely it is that he or she will tell a couple whose reproductive organs are intact, however diseased or damaged they may appear to be, that they will never have a child. Every doctor in infertility work can quote examples of couples whose chances of conceiving have seemed absolutely hopeless, but who, some months or years later, have proudly produced a child. Nevertheless, there can come a point at the end of infertility investigations where the informed opinion of the doctor can only confirm that the prospects for conception are extremely bleak indeed, and that the couple should try to adjust to the idea.

As you can imagine, the infertility investigations and attempts to produce conception with the various treatments described can stretch out over a very long period—two, three or even more years is not uncommon. Some couples will have undergone investigation in two or more centres. This is a very long time for any woman or man to have to deal with a personal problem of this magnitude, especially in the face of the persistent enquiries and occasional indirect remarks from family and friends about the long-awaited 'happy event'. As the prospect of fertility becomes more remote many couples become frustrated if their doctor's attitude is 'don't give up' and when the final crunch comes, and they are told what is by then the obvious, their reaction is often one of relief. Much of the inevitable disappointment will have come and gone already, long before the doctor finally admits to them (and himself) the unlikelihood of conception.

Calling a halt

In many gynaecological outpatient clinics in district and teaching hospitals couples passing through their series of investigations are often handed down to increasingly junior staff. In some cases a fresher approach is an advantage, especially if the senior doctor is rather old-fashioned in his methods and attitudes, but in most instances the juniors are less likely to give a considered opinion and call a halt, or at least give an indication that conception is improbable. The registrars and house officers who staff these clinics rotate appointments frequently and couples often have to deal with a different doctor at each visit.

Fortunately, many hospitals are now establishing separate infertility clinics with more permanent and experienced staff, but in the majority of situations infertile couples must compete in general clinics with other problems such as heavy periods, premenstrual tension, cancer and, sad to say, a large number of unwanted pregnancies. The demand for infertility investigations and treatment frequently outstrips capacity and in many areas waiting times, even for first visits, may be outrageously prolonged—many months and even years.

Gynaecologists and other infertility specialists, on the whole, tend to be fairly cheerful people, anxious to help, and, being friendly and good natured, they like a happy ending to a story as much as the next person. They will tend to delay announcing failure, and may subconsciously try to keep a couple's hopes alive too long. It is therefore a good idea for a couple frustrated at the end of a long period of investigations and treatment, to book an appointment with the consultant in charge of their case and ask fairly and squarely, 'Having seen all the results of our investigations and treatments, what, in your experience, and honest opinion, is the chance of our conceiving?' A direct letter to him or her is much more useful than a telephone call and will allow the consultant plenty of time to look through your notes and results at leisure before coming to an eventual opinion. The consultant can also discuss the alternatives available and referral, if necessary, to other centres, in addition to the prospects of AID, IVF, adoption etc. This will often clear the air and refresh a frustrated and disappointed couple.

Remaining childless If you have been reasonably assured that, for various reasons, conception is unlikely, there are various choices available. The obvious but often forgotten option is to stay childless and get on with life. In our overpopulated world many couples (whether potentially fertile or not) are finding the choice not to have children increasingly easy to make. The opportunities for women especially to pursue full-time career prospects, which some consider incompatible with motherhood, are also increasing rapidly. Each year a surprisingly large number of couples who have no children is requesting sterilization procedures, and doctors are responding to this change in attitude and are performing them. It may be that in the future having more than two children will be considered as anti-social as smoking in public places.

I do not offer these comments as a crumb of chilly comfort to the childless. There is a growing realization in the world that the problems of overpopulation, with the associated starvation and low standards of living, must be met by voluntary family planning methods rather than relying upon the old systems of population control—war, disease and famine. One slight regret is that the sectors of society which are consciously limiting their reproduction are a diminishing proportion of the population, whereas the proportion continuing to produce large families is increasing.

Despite these considerations, the average couple anxious to conceive are likely to be bitterly disappointed if fertility is denied them. They need time and support to overcome their loss, to readjust their lives and their relationships with each other, and with their families and friends. Sorting out the stress and any feelings of guilt and blame if one partner appears 'responsible' for the problem, and perhaps reappraising religious attitudes, will not happen in an outpatient consulting room in five or ten minutes. Above all, it is not a time for rash decisions.

There are several organizations to help the childless. In the United Kingdom the National Association for the Childless (NAC) (318 Summer Lane, Birmingham B19 3RL), was started in 1976 by Peter and Diane Houghton, who have written about their experiences of childlessness in a small booklet published by the Birmingham Settlement (a Government sponsored organization founded in 1899 to provide a place where cultural, moral and physical welfare could be enhanced) which supports NAC.

Helpful organizations

NAC has produced a large group of interested people to encourage the formation of local self-help groups throughout the country, and to determine policy at national level. NAC produces a regular newsletter giving information on new developments, reviews, letters from members and details of NAC activities. They can also put members in touch, if they wish, with others in their area with similar concerns and frequently help with counselling, if required, on adoption and fostering.

Meeting other childless couples and reading about their experiences and how they overcame their problems (or did not, as the case may be) can help the infertile couple to readjust to their emotional situation with mutual discussion and understanding. With many other problems in life one's parents are obvious providers of help and support; but although they may be supportive, by definition they may be unable to empathize fully. Childless couples should not hesitate to discuss their problem openly and frequently between themselves, and to read and hear of the experiences of others in a similar situation. Contacting the local branch of the Marriage Guidance Council may be of help. Their counsellors are trained to help couples face the strains in their relationship, whatever the reasons.

Inadequate or overstretched National Health Service facilities, lack of continuity in care, inconvenience or unsympathetic approaches may lead an infertile couple to

Private treatment

consider private treatment. I have already discussed this in relation to IVF (see p. 142), but all forms of infertility treatment can be obtained privately. Consultation fees, costs of operations and the costs of accommodation in private nursing homes and clinics vary greatly throughout the country. As with most commodities, costs tend to be higher in the big cities, where overheads and other expenses may be higher than in provincial towns. The most expensive specialist may not, however, be the best.

Your family doctor may well advise you and make helpful recommendations, as well as providing a referral letter. As infertility investigations are very personal it is wise to select a practitioner in whom you feel some kind of trust can be placed. If after the initial consultations you are getting 'bad vibrations' then it is better to cut one's losses and choose someone else. It is well worth discussing the cost of any proposed treatment at the beginning to avoid misunderstandings later.

In the United Kingdom, as in many countries, private patient insurance schemes operate, and like most insurance companies they insure against future risks, which are not known for certain, but whose odds are calculable. The situation presents one or two clear facts amongst the complexities. If a couple are infertile and then register with a private patients' scheme and declare their infertility, the proposed insurance will probably exclude infertility treatment. If they do not declare their infertility at the time of commencing the insurance they are performing a dishonest act of nondisclosure, easily discovered by a few company enquiries, which will invalidate any insurance.

It would be possible, however, for an unmarried man to insure himself with a private health plan, subsequently marry and find himself or his wife infertile and the necessary private treatment would probably be allowed under his scheme. You must check with the company concerned before embarking upon any treatment as you may find you will not be reimbursed. Some private patients are uninsured and prefer to have private investigations and treatment rather than, say, an expensive holiday.

To act as a guide only the British United Provident Association Limited issued in 1986 the following suggested surgical fee maximums to cover both payments to surgeons and anaesthetists:

Shirodkar suture, insertion and removal	Class: Intermediate	£306
Myomectomy	Class: Major	£538
Laparoscopy	Class: Intermediate	£306
Endometrium biopsy	Class: Minor	£156
Salpingostomy	Class: Major	£538
Salpingostomy (both tubes)	Class: Major plus	£661
Hysterosalpingogram	Class: Minor	£156

However, the cost of private hospital beds has increased in the last few years and continues to do so; the daily charge in private hospitals or private accommodation in NHS hospitals runs currently at between £150 and £250 per day.

In addition operating theatre fees, the cost of drugs, dressings and consultation fees must be added.

Adoption and fostering

Adoption is a legal process in which the rights and duties of the natural parents are permanently transferred by a court. Legal adoption began in England and Wales in 1926 and in Scotland in 1930 with the first adoption Acts. There was a further Act in 1958 and this has been amended by the 1975 Childrens Act. The adopted child takes the new parents' name, inherits from them and loses all legal ties to his or her family of birth. Anyone under the age of 18 who is unmarried can be adopted.

Fostering or boarding out does not involve a legal process and is a means of providing family care for a child who cannot be with his or her own parents. Often the aim is to enable the child to return eventually to his or her real parents. Foster parents may be paid allowances for maintenance, clothing etc.; adoptive parents are not paid but are entitled to child benefit. Social service departments are now heavily involved in adoption, and most fostering is organized by them. There are approximately 42 registered voluntary adoption societies in England and Wales and five in Scotland. The 1975 Act made it illegal for private placements for adoption to be made by the mother or third party, except when the proposed adopter is a relative of the child.

Over the past decade the number of babies available for adoption has declined dramatically. In England and Wales in 1968 there were 24,831 children adopted and in 1981 there were only 9,284, and of these only 3,270 were illegitimate children adopted by strangers of which only 2,211 were under the age of one year. The process of decline was hastened by changes introduced by the 1975 Act which reduced the number of adoption orders granted to step-parents. However, adoption by one or both natural parents still accounted for 54 per cent of all adoptions in 1981. Greater tolerance by society of birth out of wedlock and single parenthood, along with wider availability of contraception and legal abortions, is primarily responsible. Supply has increasingly failed to meet demand, especially for little babies.

The purpose of adoption

With this change in numbers in recent years has come a change in attitude about the purpose of adoption. Whereas in the past the supply of babies and children for adoption may have met the needs of childless couples, the attitude is now that the purpose of adoption is to find the best possible home for the child. The time for a couple to seek adoption is probably not immediately after a doctor has told them there is no hope. A period of readjustment and settling down to the idea may help before application is made to adopt. In addition to the normal responsibilities of parenthood, adoptive parents also have the task of explaining to the child about his or her origins. Adopted people are entitled to obtain their original birth certificate once they are 18 years of age and to trace their natural parents, but in practice very few do—two per thousand according to one study in Scotland.

Many adopted children nowadays are in the older age group, many have handicaps or come from socially deprived backgrounds and offer even greater problems and challenges which must be faced and overcome.

Social service departments and registered agencies have the difficult task of assessing potential adoptive parents, and their attitudes and criteria occasionally may vary somewhat. They have to think of the future as well as the present. They need to plan for the time beyond the short space of babyhood—parenthood lasts a lifetime. It is not surprising that many couples find it easier to consider AID, or even in vitro fertilization (IVF) if applicable, rather than adoption.

The British Agencies for Adoption and Fostering (11 Southwark Street, London SE1 1RQ), will send their most helpful leaflets on the subjects on receipt of a large stamped addressed envelope. 'Adoption—some questions answered', 'Foster care: some questions answered', 'Meeting children's needs through adoption and fostering', 'Talking about origins—an open letter to adoptive parents', are some of the titles. They also publish an annual review and a quarterly journal. They have centres in Wales (7 Park Grove, Cardiff CF1 3BJ), Scotland (23 Castle Street, Edinburgh EH2 3DN), the South West (9a Stokes Croft, Bristol BS1 3PL), the North (Ellison Place, Newcastle upon Tyne, NE1 8XS), and, finally, in the North West (Cranford Lodge, Bexton Road, Knutsford, Cheshire).

Adoption and fertility

Adoption has occasionally been regarded as a fertility charm since following adoption parents seem to be more likely to conceive themselves. An explanation for this apparent phenomenon is that in some couples conception is simply delayed for many years and that those couples who conceive after adopting a child probably would have done so anyway. This widely held view was tested in California. Of 1,201 couples who registered in an infertility clinic during the period 1963 to 1977, 76 were known at registration not to be at risk of pregnancy, either because an undiagnosed pregnancy existed (58 couples) or because of an untreatable condition which rendered the couple sterile (in 18). An additional 232 patients were lost to follow-up after registration. Of the 895 couples remaining, 370 (41 per cent) conceived and 525 did not. At some time after registration 128 (14 per cent) adopted. Of these adoptive couples 41 (32 per cent) conceived subsequently. The conclusion of this study was that on statistical grounds subsequent fertility was not improved by adoption. However, persistent but often anecdotal reports of women conceiving soon after adoption following many years of infertility make statistical analysis and probability tables seem too glib. The debate continues.

Surrogacy

The term surrogate, a word derived from Latin and in use even in Tudor times, means a person appointed to act in place of another. A surrogate mother is one who bears a child for another woman. There is no doubt that surrogate motherhood is a very old practice. Relations and even friends of infertile women have, throughout history, given their babies, and indeed there have been many instances when uncles and aunts have adopted nephews and nieces. Surrogacy is complicated by genetic paternity, that is to say, the man who provides the spermatozoa. This can be the partner of the surrogate mother, the partner of the infertile woman (by sexual intercourse or by artificial insemination) or even donor sperm if both recipient partners are infertile.

The whole subject throws into question what motherhood really means; new terms have been coined to describe each state. There are the 'biological' mother in whose womb the baby grows, and the 'social' mother who brings up the child. A new concept is now possible—by in vitro fertilization it is possible to insert the embryo of another couple into a surrogate mother's womb. The surrogate mother would have no genetic input into the baby but would give it birth.

The biological aspects are easy to understand—problems arise from the moral and legal standpoints.

Moral aspects of surrogacy

The word mother is very old—words sounding like mother—modor, modar, mater—have been found throughout Europe and Asia. The Oxford English Dictionary defines 'mother' as 'a woman who has given birth to a child, a female parent', but also adds, significantly, 'a woman who exercises control like that of a mother, or who is looked up to as a mother'.

Is motherhood the biological act of giving birth or is it the nurturing of the child to adolescence and adulthood? Must it be both? Is it morally right for the biological mother to give a child to a social mother? If after having given the baby away what if she subsequently wants it back? Has she any rights, morally or legally, over the child in later life? Can she see the child? Should she see the child grow up? Should the child be told of his or her 'biological' mother? Opinion on the morality of surrogacy is divided.

Many would feel that surrogacy is immoral, but speaking in a debate in the House of Lords in 1986 the Bishop of Ripon said, 'I would not want to claim that the concensus [against] extends to the total banning of surrogacy . . . indeed, even in the Church there are those who believe that it may be right and proper that a woman should offer in loving service the use of her womb to someone who is close to her.'

Legal aspects

In 1985, in a rather hasty manner and almost as an emergency measure, the Government introduced legislation to outlaw commercial surrogacy. This was in response to fears of surrogate agencies currently operating in North America setting up organizations in this country to provide mothers willing to bear a surrogate pregnancy for an infertile couple for a set fee.

The Warnock Committee made some recommendations concerning surrogacy but as yet these have not been made part of any legislation. In 1986 the Earl of Halsbury put forward a private member's Bill to incorporate into the original Act several amendments suggested by Lord Denning, the former Master of the Rolls. These sought to introduce legislation that would 'be sufficiently wide to render criminally liable the actions of professionals and others who knowingly assist in the establishment of a surrogate pregnancy'.

The Government is likely to continue its neutral stance on any future legislation, since Parliament and the people, as well as many members of religious organizations, are divided on the issue.

The medical facts of surrogacy

So back to medical facts. Using IVF it is now technically possible for a woman who has at least one functioning ovary but no uterus, say from previous surgery, or who has perhaps suffered repeated miscarriages, to have an ovum removed from her ovary. This could then be fertilized by her partner's spermatozoa and the resulting embryo could be implanted into a surrogate mother's uterus, and nine months later produce a child which is genetically derived from the infertile couple . . . who will, no doubt, call the woman who washes, clothes and feeds him or her 'mother'.

And finally

I hope this book has been useful in piloting you through the difficult waters of infertility investigations and treatments. Fortunately, many of you will have dropped out of the passage by conceiving a child before exhausting the means that modern medicine has to offer. If you have been lucky, I hope your attitude towards those who are still childless has become more understanding. If you have reached the end of investigations and are told that your cot is likely to remain empty, I hope the comments and suggestions in this book will help you adjust to your childlessness, viewing it with reasoned resignation. I also hope the depth with which I have dealt with certain problems and techniques has intrigued you and not confused you. By your enhanced knowledge of the problems, I hope you can come to terms with them better and achieve an improved understanding of what your doctor can and cannot do. We look to the future, where developments in infertility work are really exciting. The past decade has seen great advances and we hope that the next ten years are as helpful.

In the book of Genesis it says, 'And Isaac prayed unto the Lord for his wife because she was barren; and the Lord granted his prayer and Rebeckah his wife conceived.'

I hope your prayers are answered too.

Useful Addresses

Helpful organisations

Albany Trust, 32 Shaftesbury Avenue, London, W1V 8E Tel. 01-734 5588 Counselling for socio-sexual problems

Association of British Adoption Agencies, 4 Southampton Row, London, WC2B 4AA

British Agencies for Adoption and Fostering, 11 Southwark Street, London, SE1 1RQ Tel. 01-407 8800

British Diabetic Association, 10 Queen Anne Street, London, W1 Tel. 01-323 1531

Child – for infertile people, Dorothy Bull, Farthings, Gaunts Road, Paulett, Somerset

Family Planning Association, 27–35 Mortimer Street, London, W1N 7RJ Tel. 01-636 7866

Foresight: The Association for Pre-conceptual Care, The Old Vicarage, Church Lane, Witley, Godalming, Surrey Tel. 042879 4500

Genetic counselling, your GP has a list issued by DHSS

Health Education Council, 78 New Oxford Street, London, WC1A 1AH Tel. 01-631 0930

Help After Miscarriage, Miss Lynn Langendoer, Whiteleafe, 78 Ashdown Avenue, Farnborough, Hants. GU14 7DW

King's Fund Centre, 126 Albert Street, London, NW1 7NE Tel. 01-267 6112/9 Keeps lists of patient-help groups and societies

Marriage Guidance Council, 76a New Cavendish Street, London, W1 Tel. 01-580 1087

Miscarriage Association, 18 Stoneybrook Close, W. Bretton, Wakefield, W. Yorks. WF4 47P Tel. 092 485518 Sec. Mrs Kathryn Ladley

National Association for the Childless, 318 Sumner Lane, Birmingham, B19 3RL Tel. 021-359 4887/2113

National Marriage Guidance Clinic, Herbert Grey College, Little Church Street, Rugby, Warwickshire, CV21 3AP. Tel. 0788 73241

The Patients' Association, Room 33, 18 Charing Cross Road, London, WC2 Tel. 01-240 0671

Stillbirths and Neonatal Deaths Association (SANDS), Argyle House, 29–31 Euston Road, London, NW1 2S6 Tel. 01-833 2851

IVF units
(P = private clinic   NHS = National Health Service clinic)

Professor Newton, Department of Obstetrics and Gynaecology, Queen Elizabeth Hospital, Birmingham (P/NHS)

Mr M. Hull, IVF Unit, Bristol Maternity Hospital, Level D (O & G), Bristol (P/NHS)

Mr P. Steptoe, Bourn Hall Clinic, Bourn, Nr. Cambridge (P)

Dr. J. Mills, Department of Reproductive Medicine, Ninewells Hospital, Dundee (P/NHS)

Professor Beard, Department of Obstetrics and Gynaecology, The Royal Infirmary, Edinburgh (P/NHS)

Professor M. C. McNaughton, The University Department of Obstetrics and Gynaecology, Glasgow (P/NHS)

Mr D. K. Edmonds, IVF Unit, Chelsea Hospital for Women, Dovehouse Street, London, SW3 6LT (P/NHS)

Mr R. Winston, IVF Unit, Hammersmith Hospital, Ducane Road, London, W2 (P/NHS)

Professor S. Campbell, IVF Unit, Department of Obstetrics and Gynaecology, King's College Hospital, Denmark Hill, London, SE5 (P/NHS)

Mr J. Studd, IVF and GIFT Unit, Lister Hospital, Chelsea Bridge Road, London, SW1W 8RH (P)

Professor R. Shaw, Academic Department of Obstetrics and Gynaecology, Royal Free Hospital, Pond Street, London, NW3 2QG (P/NHS)

Mr M. Setchells, IVF Unit, St Bartholomews Hospital, East Smithfield, London, EC1 (P/NHS)

Dr B. Mason, The Hallam Medical Centre, 77 Hallam Street, London, W1N 5LR (P)

Mr I. Craft, IVF Unit, Wellington Humana Hospital, St John's Wood, London, NW1 (P)

Manchester Fertility Services, BUPA Hospital, Whalley Range, Manchester, M16 8AJ (P)

Mr B. Lieberman, Regional IVF Unit, St Marys Hospital, Whitworth Park, Manchester, M13 (P/NHS)

Professor M. Symons, IVF Unit, Department of Gynaecology, Queens Medical Building, Nottingham (P/NHS)

Glossary

abortifacient an instrument, drug, or other substance that provokes abortion.

abortion the loss of a fetus from the uterus before it can survive independently. When an abortion is deliberately provoked by doctors, it is known as an *induced abortion, therapeutic abortion* or *termination of pregnancy.* When it occurs naturally it is known as a *spontaneous abortion,* or a *miscarriage.*

acute a term used to describe an illness, infection, etc., that is of quick onset; sudden and of short duration, as opposed to **chronic**—neither term necessarily implies severity.

adhesions bands of scar tissue which bind organs together, they tend to form after infection or operations.

adrenal glands two small glands situated one on top of each kidney; they secrete several vital **hormones**, including some sex hormones.

adrenal hyperplasia the excessive production of adrenal hormones by an enlarged adrenal gland; it may be part of **Cushing's syndrome.**

agglutinin a substance that causes agglutination (clumping); agglutinins are sometimes found in the seminal fluid causing spermatozoa to clump together, reducing the man's fertility.

amenorrhoea the absence of menstrual periods.

amniotic fluid the liquid which surrounds the developing fetus in the uterus.

ampulla the part of the Fallopian tube nearest the ovary, where it becomes wider and bulbous.

androgens male sex hormones. Synthetic forms are sometimes used in male infertility therapy in an attempt to encourage sperm production.

anovulatory where ovulation does not occur, as in, e.g., an *anovulatory menstrual cycle.*

anteflexion a position of the uterus, in which the top of the organ is angled forwards. Compare **anteversion, retroversion.**

anteversion the common position of the uterus in the pelvis, in which the uterus is tipped forward (anteverted).

antibody a substance produced in the body to help attack foreign substances such as harmful bacteria or viruses. In some men and women antibodies are formed against spermatozoa. By neutralizing the spermatozoa, they cause infertility.

antigen any substance that causes the body to produce antibodies against it.

arrhenoblastoma a rare tumour of the ovary which may prevent ovulation from occurring by secreting male sex hormones.

artificial insemination the injection of seminal fluid into a woman's vagina, using a syringe, in order to produce a pregnancy.

azoospermia failure to produce spermatozoa; a man whose seminal fluid contains no spermatozoa is said to be *azoospermic.*

bicornuate uterus an abnormality of the uterus, the result of incomplete development before birth. Bicornuate means 'two-horned'.

biopsy removal of a small sample of tissue from the body for laboratory examination; examples are **endometrial biopsy, testicular biopsy,** and ovarian biopsy.

biphasic pattern the typical pattern recorded on a woman's monthly temperature chart, where the temperature rises by about 0.5°C (1°F) after ovulation occurs in the middle of the menstrual cycle and remains raised until menstrual bleeding starts.

blastocyst the fertilized ovum after a few day's development, at around the time it attaches itself to the wall of the uterus. At this stage it is a hollow spherical shape. Compare **morula.**

blighted ovum term used to describe a fertilized ovum that fails to develop properly after implanting into the uterus and is aborted spontaneously (miscarried).

broad ligament the fold of tissue surrounding the uterus and Fallopian tubes.

capacitation term used to describe a series of chemical changes to spermatozoa which enable them to fertilize the ovum. These changes occur as the spermatozoa pass through the plug of mucus in the cervix (neck of the uterus) and the rest of the female reproductive tract.

catheter a thin hollow tube for draining parts of the body, such as one inserted into the bladder to drain out all the urine before laparoscopy.

cauterize destroy or coagulate by applying heat; one method of sterilizing a woman is to block the Fallopian tubes by cauterizing them (*cautery*, or *diathermy*).

cervical mucus the mucus secreted by the cervix. The amount and thickness varies during the menstrual cycle, being most plentiful and thinnest at the time of ovulation. The cervical mucus plays an important role in fertilization: the spermatozoa must pass through it to reach the ovum, and as they do so important chemical changes occur (**capacitation**).

cervical os the opening of the cervix.

cervicitis inflammation of the cervix. It may be caused by bacterial or fungal infections. Cervicitis can alter the consistency of the cervical mucus, thereby causing temporary infertility.

cervix the neck of the uterus (womb).

chronic term used to describe an infection or illness that develops slowly and runs a long course; the opposite of **acute.**

cilia hairlike projections from the cells lining the Fallopian tubes which may play a part in guiding the ovum from the ovary to the uterus.

clitoris part of the external sexual organs of a woman, a small highly sensitive protuberance at the front of the vulva. During sexual excitement it becomes erect and stimulation can produce an orgasm.

clomiphene citrate a fertility drug, i.e., one which induces ovulation. It acts by causing the pituitary gland to release hormones which stimulate the ovaries to release an ovum.

combined factor infertility term used to describe a failure to conceive which is due not to a problem in either the man or the woman alone but to one which arises as a result of interaction between the two; it normally refers to failure of the man's spermatozoa to survive in the woman's vagina, perhaps because of the presence of antibodies or because the mucus secreted by the cervix is too acid.

conceptus the product of conception: the fertilized ovum, or at a later stage of development, the embryo or fetus, together with the placenta and other membranes.

cornua the horns of the uterus: the regions at the top where the Fallopian tubes enter the uterus.

corpus luteum the 'yellow body' which forms from the ovarian follicle after an ovum has been released; it secretes hormones necessary to sustain the growth of the ovum if it is fertilized.

cryopreservation preservation by freezing; spermatozoa can be frozen and stored for later use in artificial insemination.

curettage the process of scraping, e.g., of the inside of the uterus, with an instrument known as a curette. It is often performed after a miscarriage to ensure that no tissue remains behind.

cyst an abnormal accumulation of fluid, fat, or semisolid tissue in the body bounded by a capsule—a lump. One type of cyst which can affect fertility is an **ovarian cyst**, i.e. cyst on the ovary.

danazol a hormone used in the treatment of endometriosis

diabetes mellitus (usually known simply as diabetes) a disturbance of the body's metabolism of sugar caused by a failure of the pancreas to produce the hormone insulin, or an inability of the body to respond to normal insulin production. It affects fertility in both men and women

diathermy an electrical method of applying heat to parts of the body, often used to sterilize women by destroying a portion of the Fallopian tubes.

dilatation and curettage dilatation of the cervix and curettage of the uterus; a minor surgical procedure in which the opening of the cervix is dilated (widened) by passing through it rods of increasing size, and the lining of the uterus scraped using a small spoonlike instrument called a curette. Also known as **D & C.**

dysmenorrhoea painful menstruation; period pains.

dilator any device used to widen a body opening.

dyspareunia painful sexual intercourse (usually meaning pain or discomfort experienced by a woman during penetration of the vagina by a man's penis).

ectopic pregnancy a dangerous condition in which a fertilized ovum attaches itself to the lining of the Fallopian tube and begins to develop there instead of migrating to the uterus. Rarely, ectopic pregnancies may occur in other parts of the abdominal cavity.

ejaculation the act of emitting seminal fluid from the penis at orgasm.

embryo a baby at an early stage of its development in the uterus (up to about six weeks). After six weeks an unborn baby is called a **fetus.**

endocrine glands the ductless or hormone-secreting glands of the body, including the adrenal glands, pancreas, pituitary gland, ovaries, testes, thyroid and parathyroid glands.

endocrinologist a doctor who specializes in the study of **hormones,** hormonal diseases, and malfunctions, and the use of hormones in treatment.

endometrial biopsy a small sample of the endometrium (lining of the uterus) removed by curettage for examination under a microscope. The appearance of the endometrium can indicate whether ovulation has occurred.

endometriosis a condition in which abnormal growths of endometrial cells (the cells lining the uterus) appear outside the uterus in other places in the pelvis. It may cause infertility.

endometrium the glandular lining of the uterus.

enzyme a substance which acts as a catalyst in bodily processes—i.e., which regulates biochemical reactions inside the body.

epididymis a thin tube on top of the testis which connects the sperm-producing parts of the testis to the vas deferens; mature spermatozoa are stored in the epididymis.

ERPC abbreviation for Evacuation of Retained Products of Conception.

extracorporeal fertilization fertilization of an ovum outside the body; the technique of removing a ripe ovum from a woman's body, fertilizing it by mixing it with spermatozoa and injecting it into the woman's uterus. More often known as **in vitro fertilization (IVF).**

Fallopian tube the tube connecting each ovary to the uterus; it transports the ovum, after release by the ovary, to the uterus.

fetus an unborn baby after about eight weeks' development. Before that time it is known as an **embryo.**

fibroids benign tumours of the uterus, also known as *myomata*. They may distort the shape of the uterus to an extent where it cannot support a pregnancy. They can be removed surgically (**myomectomy**).

fibrosis the formation of scar tissue, for example **adhesions.**

fimbriae the finger-like projections, or fronds, at the ends of the Fallopian tubes near the ovaries. They guide the ovum into the Fallopian tube after its release from the ovary.

fimbriectomy a rarely used method of female sterilization in which the **fimbriae** are removed.

follicle–stimulating hormone (FSH) a hormone secreted by the pituitary gland. In women it stimulates the growth of the **ovarian follicle,** or ripening of the egg. In men it regulates the production of spermatozoa. It is used in infertility therapy to induce ovulation or in an attempt to improve sperm production.

fundus the upper region of the uterus, furthest from the cervix.

gas gangrene a form of gangrene (death of an area of body tissue), caused by infection with the bacterium *Clostridium*, which may occur after an incomplete abortion or miscarriage.

GIFT Gamete Intra-Fallopian Transfer: the technique of fertilization within the Fallopian tube.

gonadotrophins hormones which stimulate the sex glands, for example **follicle–stimulating hormone** and **luteinizing hormone.**

gynaecology the branch of medicine concerned with the treatment of disorders of the female reproductive system, including infertility.

heparin an anticoagulant (substance which prevents the clotting of blood).

hernia the protusion of part of the intestines through a weak spot in the wall of the abdominal cavity, normally requiring an operation to repair the defect.

hormone a chemical substance, secreted into the bloodstream by the endocrine glands, that controls the rate of bodily processes by stimulating other glands or organs.

human chorionic gonadotrophin (HCG) a hormone produced by the placenta during pregnancy and excreted in the urine. It is the substance detected in many pregnancy tests. It can be extracted from the urine of pregnant women and used in conjunction with **human menopausal gonadotrophin** to induce ovulation in women who are not ovulating.

human menopausal gonadotrophin (HMG) term used to describe **follicle–stimulating hormone** extracted from the urine of post-menopausal women. Together with **human chorionic gon-**

adotrophin, it is used in infertility therapy to induce ovulation. The urine of women at, or just after, the menopause contains large amounts of follicle stimulating hormone released by the pituitary in an attempt to provoke the release of an ovum from the ovaries, which are no longer functioning.

human pituitary gonadotrophin (HPG) term used to describe **follicle-stimulating hormone** obtained from pituitary glands of cadavers for use in infertility therapy. **Human menopausal gonadotrophin** is easier to obtain and is therefore more widely used.

hydrosalpinges accumulations of fluid in the Fallopian tubes, causing them to bulge. The cause is blockage at the ends of the tubes nearest the ovaries.

hydrotubation the process of passing water through the cervix to wash out the Fallopian tubes, for example after surgical repair of the tubes.

hymen a thin membrance partially covering the entrance to the vagina in virgins, also called 'maidenhead'.

hypoplastic uterus a severely undersized uterus.

hypospadias an abnormality of the penis in which the urethra (the tube which carries urine out of the body) opens on the underside of the penis and not at the tip. *Epispadias* is a similar abnormality where the opening of the urethra is along the top of the penis.

hypothalamus a centre in the brain lying directly above the pituitary gland. The hypothalamus controls many bodily functions, and plays an important part in regulating the hormone output of the pituitary gland; it also monitors the level of hormones and other substances circulating in the bloodstream.

hysterosalpingogram (HSG) an x-ray picture of the cavity of the uterus and the Fallopian tubes obtained by passing a radiopaque fluid (one which is opaque to x-rays) through the cervix.

immune system the body's defences against infection. The most important components are the white blood cells, which attack invading organisms such as bacteria and viruses, either directly or by producing **antibodies**.

implantation the process in which the fertilized ovum attaches itself to the lining of the uterus, which supports and nourishes it.

impotence the inability, whether temporary or permanent, of a man to produce or sustain an erection of the penis.

incompetent cervix a weakened cervix that is not sufficiently strong to remain closed during pregnancy and may cause miscarriage (loss of the fetus).

insufflation (also known as Rubin's test) an old-fashioned test to determine whether the Fallopian tubes are open (patent) by passing gas through the cervix. The passage of the gas escaping from the tubes can be heard by a doctor with a stethoscope applied to the abdomen. Obstructions can also be indicated on a pressure chart.

In vitro fertilization (IVF) see **extracorporeal fertilization**.

isthmus the narrow portion of the Fallopian tubes close to the junction with the uterus.

laparoscope an instrument which is passed through the wall of the abdomen to examine internal organs, consisting of a long narrow telescope with an eyepiece at one end and a light source for illuminating the abdominal cavity.

laparoscopy the use of laparoscope to

examine internal organs.

laparotomy an incision into the abdomen.

lumen the space inside a tube in the body.

luteal phase the second half of the menstrual cycle, after ovulation has occurred, when the **corpus luteum** in the ovary secretes hormones necessary to sustain the growth of a fertilized ovum.

luteinizing hormone a hormone secreted by the pituitary gland. In women it helps to stimulate ovulation and the development of the **corpus luteum**. In men it stimulates maturation of certain cells in the testes and the secretion of male sex hormones.

lysis of adhesions cutting of adhesions (bands of scar tissue) inside the abdominal cavity.

menarche a girl's first menstrual period.

menopause the natural cessation of a woman's menstrual periods; 'change of life'.

menorrhagia heavy menstrual bleeding.

menstrual cycle the regular changes that occur on an approximately monthly cycle in the female reproductive system after puberty and before the menopause, involving the release of an ovum from the ovary, the growth of the endometrium in readiness to receive a fertilized ovum, and, if no pregnancy occurs, the loss of blood and endometrial tissue from the vagina (**menstruation**).

menstruation the loss of blood from the vagina that occurs at the end of the **menstrual cycle**.

mesterolone a male sex hormone which has been used in infertility therapy in an attempt to improve sperm production.

mittelschmerz pain experienced in the middle of the menstrual cycle.

morula the fertilized ovum after a few days' development, when it forms a solid ball of cells.

mucorrhoea abundant production of mucus; the increase in cervical mucus near the time of ovulation is known as cervical mucorrhoea.

myomectomy an operation to remove **fibroids** from the uterus.

obstetrics the branch of medicine concerned with the care of pregnant women and their babies up until childbirth and shortly after.

oestrogen the major female sex hormone (in fact, there are several different types of oestrogen) which is secreted mainly by the ovaries.

oligospermia the production of relatively low numbers of spermatozoa; a man whose fluid contains low concentrations of spermatozoa is said to be oligospermic.

orchidectomy surgical removal of a testis.

orchidopexy an operation to bring a maldescended testis down into the scrotum.

ovarian cyst a cyst growing in an ovary; most are benign, but some are malignant. They can reach a considerable size and are usually removed surgically. Sometimes multiple small cysts appear—the **polycystic ovary syndrome**.

ovarian follicle a tiny sac within the ovary containing an ovum (egg cell). During each **menstrual cycle** one ovum begins to grow and ripen; as it does so the follicle enlarges until, at **ovulation**, the follicle bursts to release the mature ovum. The **corpus luteum** develops from the follicle after release of the ovum.

ovary the female reproductive organ which secretes ova (egg cells). There are two ovaries situated one on each side of the uterus. They are each about the size of an almond in its shell. As well as producing ova they secrete sex hormones, notably oestrogen and, after ovulation, progesterone (from the **corpus luteum**).

ovulation the release of an ovum (egg cell) from an ovary. Ovulation normally occurs each month at approximately the midpoint of the menstrual cycle. Under the influence of hormones from the pituitary gland, an ovarian follicle develops and eventually releases a ripe ovum which travels down the Fallopian tube awaiting fertilization.

ovum (plural **ova**) the female reproductive cell (egg cell), which, if fertilized by a spermatozoon, will grow inside the uterus into an embryo and fetus.

pancreas an organ lying just below and behind the stomach; one of the **endocrine glands**. Among its functions is to secrete the hormone insulin, which regulates the metabolism of sugar. A deficiency of, or lack of response to, insulin leads to **diabetes mellitus**.

parasympathetic nervous system part of the autonomic nervous system, which helps with short-term control of the automatic functions of the body (breathing, heart rate, digestion, etc.). In general it opposes the action of the **sympathetic nervous system.** The parasympathetic nervous system controls, among other functions, the erection of the penis.

patent a technical word meaning open, especially when referring to the Fallopian tubes.

pelvic inflammatory disease (PID) generalized infection involving the pelvic organs, especially the ovaries and Fallopian tubes, which may result in damage to or blockage of the Fallopian tubes.

pelvis strictly speaking, the bony basin-shaped structure at the end of the spine; however the word is used loosely to mean the pelvic organs, an expression which normally refers to the female internal reproductive organs—ovaries, Fallopian tubes, and uterus.

peritoneal cavity the space within the abdomen, containing the internal organs.

pessary a device inserted into the vagina, such as a device to support or alter the position of the uterus, or a medication which will dissolve and treat localized conditions, or be absorbed into the bloodstream through the vaginal lining for generalized ones.

pituitary gland a pea-sized gland situated at the base of the brain, behind the eyes. Partly under the control of the **hypothalamus** (a structure lying directly above it), the pituitary gland secretes a variety of hormones essential for many bodily processes, including the function of the reproductive system. Two important pituitary hormones are follicle-stimulating hormone and luteinizing hormone, which regulate ovulation in women and sperm production in men.

placenta the afterbirth; the fleshy pancake-shaped organ to which the developing embryo and fetus is connected by the umbilical cord, and through which it respires and receives nourishment.

polycystic ovary syndrome a condition in which multiple small cysts appear in the ovaries; also known as the Stein-Leventhal syndrome. Women with polycystic ovaries often fail to ovulate, but ovulation can usually be restored by administering fertility drugs or by surgically removing a wedge of tissue from the ovary (wedge resection).

postcoital after coitus (sexual intercourse).

postcoital test a procedure to determine

how well a man's spermatozoa survive inside his partner's body. It consists of removing a small drop of cervical mucus from the woman's vagina a short time after intercourse has taken place and examining it under a microscope.

premature menopause a condition in which the **menopause** occurs unusually early in life, in a woman's 30s or earlier rather than the late 40s or early 50s. The cause is not fully understood.

primary infertility failure to produce a child by a couple (or by a woman or man) who have not previously produced a child.

progesterone one of the principal female sex hormones, secreted mainly by the **corpus luteum** in the ovary after ovulation has occurred. It prepares the uterus for pregnancy.

progestogen a hormone similar in effect to **progesterone.** Synthetic progestogens are used in oral contraceptives, and sometimes in the treatment of endometriosis.

prolactin a hormone secreted by the pituitary gland; its function is to stimulate the milk-secreting glands of the breast after childbirth. Abnormally high levels of prolactin can cause infertility in women by interfering with ovulation; it is being investigated as a possible factor in male infertility.

proliferative phase the stage of the menstrual cycle which follows the cessation of menstrual bleeding, during which the endometrium grows (proliferates) in preparation for a possible pregnancy.

prostaglandins hormone-like substances found in the body and which have a powerful effect on the blood vessels and metabolism, and especially on the uterus. They are implicated as a possible cause of infertility in women with endometriosis.

prostatectomy removal of all or part of the prostate gland, usually performed to relieve obstruction of the urinary passage caused by enlargement of the gland in late life or by a tumour.

prostate gland a gland situated at the base of the bladder in men; it surrounds the urethra—the tube which carries urine and seminal fluid out of the penis—and is about the size and shape of a walnut. Its secretions form part of the **seminal fluid.**

prostatitis inflammation of the prostate gland, usually as a result of infection with bacteria. Prostatitis sometimes appears to cause the formation of antisperm **antibodies;** it can be treated with antibiotics.

prosthesis any artificial device used to replace a part of the body, whether for functional purposes or for appearance. Examples are false teeth, artificial limbs, and, in infertility work, implants or other devices used to achieve erection of the penis in cases of impotence.

psychosexual counselling help and advice given by trained personnel to assist overcoming sexual problems such as premature ejaculation, impotence of psychological origin, frigidity, vaginal spasm, etc.

radiographer a technician who takes and processes x-ray photographs or films.

radiologist a doctor skilled in analysing and interpreting x-rays.

radiopaque opaque to x-rays; radiopaque substances are used to obtain an x-ray picture of a hollow area in the body. For example, if a patient swallows a 'meal' of radiopaque liquid, the outline of his stomach will show up on an x-ray film. A **hysterosalpingogram** (HSG) involves filling the uterus with a radiopaque fluid.

radiotherapy the use of radiation and radioactive substances to treat cancer.

recanalize to join up again or heal, forming a channel; term used, for example, to describe the healing of tubes such as the Fallopian tubes or the vasa deferentia after a sterilization procedure.

retrograde menstruation theory a theory to account for the development of **endometriosis** which assumes that endometrial cells, after being shed by the uterus at menstruation, find their way out of the uterus through the Fallopian tubes instead of being lost along with the menstrual blood through the vagina.

retroversion a position of the uterus, in which it is angled backwards rather than forwards in the pelvis. It occurs in approximately one in five women. Compare **anteversion, anteflexion**.

round ligaments two round strips of muscle and connective tissue that help to hold the uterus in position.

salpingitis inflammation of the Fallopian tubes caused by infection. Infection can cause blockage of the tubes, or can damage their lining, and thus cause infertility by preventing an ovum from reaching the uterus.

salpingostomy an operation to open up Fallopian tubes which are blocked at the end nearest the ovary (fimbrial end).

secretory phase the last part of the menstrual cycle, lasting about 14 days, from the time of ovulation until the beginning of menstruation, during which the lining of the uterus (**endometrium**) is ready to receive a fertilized egg.

secondary infertility infertility in a couple (or a woman or man) who have already conceived or produced a conception previously.

seminal fluid the milky-white fluid emitted from a man's penis at orgasm, consisting principally of the secretions of the prostate gland, seminal vesicles, and spermatozoa, which may number up to 500 million or more; also called *semen* or *ejaculate*.

seminal vesicles two small glands lying behind the bladder in men through which the vasa deferentia (sperm-carrying tubes) pass before joining up with the urethra. The secretions of the seminal vesicles form part of the seminal fluid.

seminalysis analysis of a man's seminal fluid to assess whether he is likely to be fertile; the important criteria are the number and quality of spermatozoa, and the presence or absence of certain other substances. Its implications may often be difficult to predict accurately.

serum progesterone test a test to measure the amount of the hormone progesterone in the blood. This can show whether a woman has ovulated because after ovulation the level of progesterone rises to prepare the body for a possible pregnancy.

speculum an instrument to allow examination of a body cavity or passage by dilating (widening) it, for example, a *vaginal speculum*.

sperm-cervical mucus contact test a test to assess whether a woman's cervical mucus is hostile to her partner's spermatozoa, in which a small quantity of mucus is removed and mixed with a drop of the man's seminal fluid. The spermatozoa's progress is examined under a microscope.

spermicide a substance that kills spermatozoa.

sterilization an operation to terminate a man's or woman's fertility. Male sterilization, known as **vasectomy**, consists of cutting and tying off the vasa deferentia (sperm-carrying tubes).

Female sterilization usually consists of blocking, cutting or destroying a small section of the Fallopian tubes.

steroids a large group of organic compounds, including many hormones and some vitamins. Steroids have important uses as anti–inflammatory drugs.

subfertility term used to describe any impairment of fertility or unusual delay in producing offspring, without implying permanent infertility.

suture a stitch to close a wound, surgical incision, etc.

sympathetic nervous system part of the autonomic nervous system. Among the functions of the sympathetic nervous system are the control of ejaculation. See also **parasympathetic nervous system**.

tamoxifen a fertility drug, i.e., one which induces ovulation. Its action is similar to that of **clomiphene citrate**.

testis (plural **testes**) the male reproductive organ which produces spermatozoa.

testosterone the principal male sex hormone, secreted mainly by the testes. It is involved in sperm production and in the development of secondary sexual characteristics.

testosterone rebound therapy a treatment sometimes used in the treatment of low sperm production. Injections of testosterone, which have the effect of suppressing sperm production, are given for a period of time in the hope that when treatment is stopped, sperm production will rise (rebound) to improved levels.

T-mycoplasma a micro-organism that is intermediate in size between a virus and a bacterium. Its role in infertility is not understood, but it has been implicated as a possible cause of recurrent miscarriage.

toxins poisonous substances produced by micro–organisms.

toxoplasma a protozoan (one-celled animal) which may infect women and occasionally cause miscarriages (spontaneous abortions). Infections of toxoplasma organisms during pregnancy may cause damage in the fetus.

thermography a diagnostic technique involving measuring the heat given off by the body; a picture, called a *thermogram*, is built up showing the different temperatures of various parts of the body as areas of different colours.

thermolysis the cutting of adhesions (bands of scar tissue inside the abdominal cavity) using an electrically heated instrument.

thyroid gland one of the **endocrine glands**, situated in the neck in front of the windpipe. The hormones it releases control the rate of metabolism (the rate at which the body consumes energy). Four smaller glands, the **parathyroid glands**, are embedded within the thyroid. Their hormones control the levels of calcium and phosphorus in the body.

Turner's syndrome a chromosomal abnormality of women in which one of the sex chromosomes is missing (giving a 45X configuration of chromosomes instead of the normal 46XX). This deficiency results in abnormal development of the ovary, which lacks most or all of its ova. Such women are infertile and may never menstruate, or their menstrual cycles cease while they are still adolescent.

ultrasound scan a technique for visualizing internal organs. High-frequency sound waves (which are inaudible) are directed at the area under examination. They are reflected back as 'echoes' which can be built up into a picture on a screen. Ultrasound can delineate some structures which do not show up on x-rays, and is also very useful for examining the pregnant uterus (x-rays are dangerous to the developing fetus).

undescended testis term used to describe a testis which, at birth, has not descended into the scrotum as normal. An operation is usually performed during childhood to bring the testis down if it fails to descend normally. Testes which did not descend properly at birth may well be associated with impaired fertility. There is also an increased risk of malignant tumours forming in undescended testes which are not brought down surgically.

unicornuate uterus an abnormality of the uterus, the result of incomplete development before birth. Unicornuate means 'having one cornua (horn)'.

urethra the passage, or tube, which carries urine from the bladder out of the body. In men it also receives the seminal fluid from the vasa deferentia and carries it out through the penis.

urologist a doctor who specializes in the treatment of disorders of the genital organs and urinary system. The urologist often investigates and treats male infertility.

uterus the womb; the muscular organ in a woman's pelvis which nourishes and protects the growing fetus during pregnancy. When not pregnant it is about the size and shape of a pear. At the upper end it branches out into the Fallopian tubes; at the lower end lies the neck of the uterus, or **cervix**. The glandular lining of the uterus, the **endometrium**, undergoes regular changes throughout the menstrual cycle.

vagina part of a woman's internal genital organs; the muscular sheath which receives a man's penis during sexual intercourse and through which a baby is expelled from the body at childbirth.
course and through which a baby is expelled from the body at childbirth.

vaginal spasm spasm of the vaginal muscles (inability to relax) during or before sexual intercourse, preventing satisfactory penetration by the penis. It is normally due to fear, inhibition, or other psychological factors.

vaginismus another name for **vaginal spasm.**

varicocele an abnormality of the network of blood vessels through the scrotum, in which veins enlarge and become tortuous (twisted). This has the effect of raising the temperature of the testes, which may impair sperm production. An operation can be performed to correct the condition.

vas deferens (plural **vasa deferentia**) the muscular tube that connects the epididymis (where spermatozoa are stored on top of the testis) to the prostate gland. At ejaculation spermatozoa are conducted along the two vasa deferentia to the prostate gland, where together with other secretions and fluids they pass into the urethra and out through the penis.

vasectomy the operation to sterilize a man, in which the two **vasa deferentia** are cut and tied back.

vasoepididymostomy an operation to remove an obstruction from blocked **vasa deferentia.**

venereal disease any disease transmitted by sexual intercourse. Some, such as **gonorrhoea** and **syphilis**, can affect fertility.

viable (1) (of a spermatozoon) able to fertilize an ovum. Once inside a woman's body, the life of spermatozoa is limited, usually to between 48 and 72 hours. (2) (of an ovum) able to be fertilized by a spermatozoon. Ova usually die about 18–24 hours after being released by the ovary. (3) (of a fetus) sufficiently well developed to be able to survive outside its mother's body (legally after 28 weeks' gestation).

vulva the external genital organs of a woman, consisting of the *labia majora* and *labia minora* (the outer and inner folds of flesh around the vaginal opening) and the **clitoris**. The opening of the urethra lies just below the clitoris.

wedge resection an operation to treat severe cases of the **polycystic ovary syndrome** in which a wedge of the ovary is removed. This sometimes restores ovarian function (i.e., ovulation).

white blood cells one of the components of the blood; their function is to defend the body against infection, and they are an important part of the **immune system**. They are larger and much less numerous than the red blood cells, whose principal function is to transport oxygen and nutrients to the body tissues.

womb the **uterus**.

zygote a fertilized ovum, or more correctly the cell resulting from the union of a spermatozoon and an ovum.

Index